AF354058

Clinical Documentation Specialist

-

The Comprehensive Guide

by

VIRUTI SHIVAN

Masters in Clinical Psychology (Major)

"In books, as in life, it's not the size or looks but the content that matters."

DISCLAIMER: The information in this book is provided for general informational purposes only and is not intended as professional advice. Although every effort has been made to ensure the accuracy and completeness of the information, the author and publisher do not assume responsibility for errors, inaccuracies, omissions, inconsistencies, or the impact of future advancements or updates in technology and information. This book is not a substitute for proper training, diagnosis, treatment, or guidance from qualified professionals. Readers are encouraged to consult experts in the relevant fields and independently verify the information when necessary. Any slights of people, places, or organizations are unintentional and purely coincidental.

Introduction

In the complex and dynamic world of healthcare, the role of clinical documentation cannot be overstated. It serves as the cornerstone of quality patient care, legal integrity, billing accuracy, and healthcare analytics. **Clinical Documentation Specialist - The Comprehensive Guide** aims to equip healthcare professionals, especially those new to the field or looking to refine their expertise, with the knowledge and skills necessary to excel in this critical role.

Clinical documentation is more than just recording patient interactions; it's about capturing a holistic view of the patient's journey through the healthcare system. This process ensures that every diagnosis, treatment, and healthcare service is accurately documented, reflecting the patient's status and the care provided. Such documentation is pivotal not only for direct patient care but also for legal protection, compliance with healthcare regulations, and the facilitation of billing processes.

The evolution of technology, particularly the adoption of Electronic Health Records (EHRs), has significantly transformed clinical documentation practices. With these changes come new challenges and opportunities for documentation specialists. This guide delves into these aspects, offering a blend of foundational knowledge, current trends, and forward-looking insights into the future of clinical documentation.

Through this comprehensive exploration, the guide aims to foster a deep understanding of the principles of effective documentation, the importance of accuracy and compliance, and the impact of documentation on patient outcomes and healthcare efficiency. It provides actionable strategies, theoretical frameworks, and practical tips to navigate the complexities of clinical documentation in today's digital age.

As we embark on this journey together, the ultimate goal of this guide is to empower you to become a more effective, efficient, and informed clinical documentation specialist. Whether you're aiming to enhance your current skills or build a foundation for a new career in healthcare documentation, this guide is your companion, offering insights and knowledge that are both deep and accessible, tailored to the needs of professionals dedicated to excellence in healthcare.

Chapter 1: The Foundations of Clinical Documentation

1.1 The Importance of Accurate Clinical Documentation

In the realm of healthcare, accurate clinical documentation serves as the backbone of quality patient care, compliance, and efficient healthcare delivery. This critical function goes beyond mere record-keeping; it is an integral component of the healthcare ecosystem that ensures patients receive timely, accurate, and effective treatment. Accurate documentation facilitates clear communication among care teams, supports billing and reimbursement processes, and aids in legal protection for healthcare providers and institutions.

The Bedrock of Patient Care

At its core, accurate clinical documentation directly impacts patient outcomes. It provides a detailed account of a patient's medical history, current condition, treatment plans, and progress notes, allowing for a comprehensive and holistic approach to patient care. This continuity of information is crucial in scenarios where multiple specialists are involved in a patient's care, ensuring that every healthcare provider has access to the same information, reducing errors, and enhancing the quality of care.

Legal and Compliance Safeguard

In the ever-evolving landscape of healthcare regulations, accurate documentation is a critical ally. It serves as evidence of the care provided, justifying the treatments and interventions undertaken. In the face of audits, legal disputes, or compliance reviews, thorough and accurate documentation can protect healthcare providers and institutions by demonstrating adherence to established guidelines, standards, and legal requirements.

Facilitator of Effective Communication

Effective communication is vital in healthcare, and clinical documentation is a primary medium through which this occurs. It allows for seamless transitions of care, whether between shifts, departments, or different healthcare facilities. Accurate documentation ensures that every healthcare provider involved in a patient's care has a clear understanding of the patient's status, treatment plan, and any other relevant information, thus minimizing miscommunications and errors.

Enhancement of Healthcare Efficiency and Billing

From an administrative perspective, accurate clinical documentation is indispensable for efficient operation and financial sustainability of healthcare services. It supports accurate coding and billing, ensuring that healthcare providers are reimbursed for the services rendered. This accuracy is essential not only for the financial health of medical practices but also for reducing the incidence of fraud and abuse in billing, a concern that continues to gain attention in healthcare systems worldwide.

Personalized Patient Care

Finally, accurate clinical documentation supports the trend towards personalized medicine. By maintaining comprehensive and detailed patient records, healthcare providers can tailor treatment plans to the individual needs of each patient. This approach leads to better patient outcomes, higher patient satisfaction, and more efficient use of healthcare resources.

In summary, the importance of accurate clinical documentation cannot be overstated. It is a fundamental aspect of healthcare that supports patient care, legal compliance, effective communication, and the operational efficiency of healthcare services. As we delve deeper into the principles of clinical documentation, it becomes evident that mastering this aspect of healthcare is crucial for anyone involved in the provision of medical services.

1.2 Understanding the Healthcare Environment

Navigating the healthcare environment requires a comprehensive understanding of its complex and multifaceted nature. This environment is characterized by its dynamic interplay between patient care, regulatory compliance, technological advancements, and the pursuit of operational efficiency. For clinical documentation specialists, grasping these elements is crucial for effectively contributing to patient care and the broader healthcare system.

Patient-Centered Care

At the heart of the healthcare environment is patient-centered care. This approach emphasizes the importance of understanding patients' needs, preferences, and values, and using that knowledge to guide all decisions. Clinical documentation plays a critical role in ensuring that every member of the healthcare team is informed about the patient's history, preferences, and treatment plans, thereby enabling a coordinated and personalized approach to care.

Regulatory Landscape

Healthcare providers operate within a regulatory framework designed to ensure patient safety, privacy, and quality of care. Laws and regulations such as the Health Insurance Portability and Accountability Act (HIPAA) in the United States set strict guidelines for the handling of patient information, including its documentation, storage, and sharing. Clinical documentation specialists must be adept at navigating these regulations to maintain compliance and protect patient rights.

Technological Advancements

Technology is a driving force in the evolution of the healthcare environment. Electronic Health Records (EHRs), telehealth, and mobile health applications are transforming how care is delivered and documented. These technologies offer opportunities to improve the accuracy and efficiency of clinical documentation but also introduce challenges related to interoperability, data security, and the learning curve for new users. Understanding these technological tools and how they integrate with clinical documentation processes is essential for specialists in this field.

Interdisciplinary Collaboration

Healthcare delivery is inherently interdisciplinary, involving a wide range of professionals from doctors and nurses to pharmacists, social workers, and beyond. Effective clinical documentation ensures that all team members have access to up-to-date, accurate information, facilitating collaboration and coordination of care. Understanding the roles and perspectives of different healthcare professionals can enhance the quality and effectiveness of clinical documentation.

Healthcare Economics and Efficiency

Economic considerations significantly influence the healthcare environment. Clinical documentation impacts the financial aspects of healthcare delivery through its role in billing, reimbursement, and resource allocation. Accurate documentation ensures that healthcare providers are fairly compensated for their services and that resources are allocated efficiently, contributing to the sustainability of healthcare systems.

Quality Improvement and Patient Safety

Finally, the healthcare environment is increasingly focused on quality improvement and patient safety. Clinical documentation is a valuable tool for tracking outcomes, identifying trends, and implementing changes to improve patient care. Specialists must understand how documentation contributes to quality improvement initiatives and patient safety efforts, using data to drive better health outcomes.

Understanding the healthcare environment is critical for clinical documentation specialists. This knowledge enables them to contribute effectively to patient care, navigate the regulatory landscape, leverage technological advancements, collaborate across disciplines, address economic challenges, and support quality improvement efforts. By appreciating the complexity and dynamism of this environment, specialists can play a pivotal role in enhancing the efficiency, quality, and safety of healthcare delivery.

1.3 Legal and Ethical Considerations in Documentation

In the healthcare sector, clinical documentation intersects significantly with legal and ethical standards, necessitating a careful balance between comprehensive patient care, privacy, and compliance with regulations. This balance is crucial in fostering trust, ensuring justice, and upholding the dignity of patients while navigating the complexities of healthcare delivery.

Legal Frameworks Guiding Documentation

Legal considerations in clinical documentation are primarily concerned with compliance with laws and regulations at both national and international levels. Key among these is the Health Insurance Portability and Accountability Act (HIPAA) in the United States, which sets the standard for protecting sensitive patient data. Similar regulations exist globally, each designed to ensure that patient information is handled securely and confidentially, and that documentation practices do not infringe on patient rights.

Documentation also plays a pivotal role in the legal process, serving as evidence in cases of malpractice or negligence. Accurate and timely entries can demonstrate adherence to standard care protocols, while gaps or inaccuracies in documentation can lead to legal vulnerabilities. It is essential for healthcare providers to be aware of the legal implications of their documentation practices, including the necessity for consent and the accurate reflection of patient interactions and care provided.

Ethical Considerations in Documentation

Ethically, clinical documentation must respect patient autonomy and confidentiality. This involves obtaining informed consent for treatments and ensuring that personal health information is shared only with those directly involved in the patient's care or as mandated by law. Ethical documentation practices also require objectivity and accuracy, free from personal bias or alteration.

Healthcare providers face ethical dilemmas when documentation intersects with patient rights. For example, how to document sensitive information that a patient does not wish to be recorded, or how to ensure the documentation reflects all aspects of care, including any errors or adverse events. The principle of non-maleficence, or "do no harm," extends to documentation practices, emphasizing the importance of accurate and honest recording to avoid harm to the patient.

Navigating Legal and Ethical Complexities

To navigate these legal and ethical considerations effectively, healthcare providers must be well-versed in relevant laws and ethical guidelines. Regular training and education on changes in legislation, privacy practices, and ethical documentation standards are essential. Moreover, institutions should establish clear policies and procedures for documentation, including protocols for handling sensitive information, correcting errors, and safeguarding against unauthorized access to patient records.

Conclusion

Legal and ethical considerations in clinical documentation are integral to the practice of medicine, reflecting the broader values of society regarding

privacy, justice, and patient care. Healthcare providers are tasked with the dual responsibility of adhering to stringent legal requirements while navigating the ethical landscape of patient interactions. Through comprehensive understanding and application of these principles, healthcare professionals can ensure their documentation practices contribute positively to patient care, uphold legal standards, and embody the ethical commitments of their profession. This dual adherence not only enhances patient trust and safety but also fortifies the healthcare system against potential legal and ethical challenges, ensuring a more robust, equitable, and compassionate delivery of care.

1.4 Exercise: 10 MCQs with Answers at the End

Test your knowledge on the foundations of clinical documentation with these multiple-choice questions (MCQs). The correct answers are provided at the end to help you assess your understanding of the topics covered in Chapter 1.

1. What is the primary purpose of clinical documentation?

   A) Billing and coding

   B) Legal protection

   C) Facilitating patient care

   D) Research purposes

2. Which law is primarily concerned with the protection of patient health information in the United States?

   A) GDPR

   B) HIPAA

   C) Affordable Care Act

   D) American Medical Association guidelines

3. Accurate clinical documentation is crucial for:

A) Ensuring patient privacy

B) Facilitating communication among healthcare providers

C) Supporting billing and reimbursement processes

D) All of the above

4. Ethical considerations in clinical documentation include all EXCEPT:

A) Objectivity in recording patient information

B) Altering documentation to protect patient privacy

C) Obtaining informed consent for treatments documented

D) Ensuring accuracy and completeness of records

5. Which of the following is NOT a direct benefit of accurate clinical documentation?

A) Reduced healthcare costs

B) Increased patient satisfaction

C) Higher rates of medication errors

D) Improved patient outcomes

6. Legal vulnerabilities in clinical documentation can arise from:

A) Timely and accurate entries

B) Gaps or inaccuracies in documentation

C) Adherence to standard care protocols

D) Compliance with HIPAA regulations

7. The principle of "do no harm" in the context of documentation emphasizes:

A) The need for comprehensive documentation

B) Accuracy and honesty in recording

C) The importance of patient confidentiality

D) All of the above

8. Effective communication through clinical documentation is vital for:

A) Ensuring continuity of care

B) Reducing the risk of legal action

C) Billing purposes

D) A and B

9. Informed consent for treatments documented is primarily related to:

A) Legal considerations

B) Ethical considerations

C) Both legal and ethical considerations

D) Neither legal nor ethical considerations

10. A key legal requirement for clinical documentation includes:

A) Regular deletion of outdated patient information

B) Sharing patient information with all hospital staff

C) Secure handling of patient records

D) Use of patient information for marketing purposes

Answers:

1. C) Facilitating patient care

2. B) HIPAA

3. D) All of the above

4. B) Altering documentation to protect patient privacy

5. C) Higher rates of medication errors

6. B) Gaps or inaccuracies in documentation

7. D) All of the above

8. D) A and B

9. C) Both legal and ethical considerations

10. C) Secure handling of patient records

Chapter 2: Principles of Effective Documentation

2.1 Clarity, Conciseness, and Coherence

In the intricate landscape of healthcare, the principles of clarity, conciseness, and coherence stand as foundational pillars in the realm of clinical documentation. These principles not only facilitate effective communication among healthcare providers but also ensure that documentation fulfills its role in patient care, legal compliance, and healthcare management efficiently.

Clarity: Illuminating Patient Care

Clarity in clinical documentation involves the use of straightforward and unambiguous language to describe patient encounters, diagnoses, treatments, and outcomes. This principle ensures that all healthcare providers, regardless of their specialty or level of expertise, can understand the patient's medical history and care plan without misinterpretation. Clarity eliminates confusion, reducing the risk of errors in patient care. It involves avoiding medical jargon when possible or clearly defining terms that may not be universally understood, thereby making the information accessible to all members of the healthcare team, including patients.

Conciseness: The Essence of Efficiency

Conciseness in documentation means conveying necessary information as briefly as possible without omitting critical details. This principle respects the time of healthcare providers and facilitates quick access to essential information, especially in urgent care situations. Conciseness helps in avoiding overly verbose notes that can bury important details under unnecessary information, making it challenging to quickly grasp a patient's status or history. Effective documentation strikes a balance, ensuring that while brevity is maintained, completeness is not compromised.

Coherence: A Seamless Narrative

Coherence in clinical documentation ensures that the information presented follows a logical flow, making it easy for anyone reading the record to follow the patient's healthcare journey. This involves organizing information in a systematic manner, using a consistent format, and linking related pieces of information in a way that makes sense. Coherence supports the continuity of care, as it allows subsequent caregivers to understand the thought processes of previous providers, the rationale behind diagnostic and treatment decisions, and the expected course of care.

Applying the Principles

To apply these principles effectively, healthcare professionals can adopt structured documentation formats such as SOAP (Subjective, Objective, Assessment, Plan) notes, which naturally guide the documentation process in a clear, concise, and coherent manner. Additionally, regular training and feedback on documentation practices can help refine these skills, ensuring that clinical records serve their purpose as efficiently as possible.

In conclusion, clarity, conciseness, and coherence are not just stylistic preferences but essential attributes of effective clinical documentation. They ensure that patient records are accurate, accessible, and actionable, supporting high-quality patient care and the smooth operation of healthcare systems. As we delve further into the principles of effective documentation, it becomes evident how these foundational attributes influence all aspects of clinical documentation, from legal compliance to patient engagement and healthcare outcomes.

2.2 The Role of Electronic Health Records (EHRs)

The advent of Electronic Health Records (EHRs) has revolutionized the landscape of clinical documentation, transforming traditional paper-based records into dynamic, digital formats. EHRs play a pivotal role in enhancing the principles of effective documentation—clarity, conciseness, and coherence—while introducing new capabilities that extend far beyond these foundational aspects. This transition to digital records has significantly impacted healthcare delivery, offering a more integrated, efficient, and patient-centered approach to medical documentation.

Enhancing Accessibility and Communication

One of the primary advantages of EHRs is the ease of access they provide. Healthcare providers can access patient records instantaneously from any location, fostering improved communication and collaboration across care teams. This instant access facilitates a more coordinated approach to patient care, allowing for real-time updates and ensuring that all members of the healthcare team are on the same page regarding patient treatment plans and outcomes.

Promoting Standardization and Quality of Care

EHRs contribute to the standardization of documentation practices through the use of templates and structured input fields. These features help in maintaining clarity and conciseness in documentation, reducing variability in how information is recorded. Standardization ensures that critical patient information is captured systematically, enhancing the quality of patient care by enabling comprehensive and accurate clinical assessments.

Supporting Decision Making and Analytics

EHRs are equipped with decision support tools that aid healthcare providers in making informed treatment decisions based on evidence-based guidelines and the patient's specific health data. These systems can alert providers to potential issues, such as drug interactions or deviations from clinical guidelines, thus improving patient safety. Additionally, the aggregation of data within EHRs supports healthcare analytics, enabling the analysis of trends, outcomes, and performance metrics that can inform quality improvement initiatives and public health strategies.

Facilitating Patient Engagement

EHRs also play a crucial role in patient engagement by providing patients with access to their health information through patient portals. This accessibility empowers patients to take an active role in their healthcare, fostering better communication between patients and providers, and enhancing patient satisfaction and adherence to treatment plans.

Addressing Challenges and Opportunities

While EHRs offer numerous benefits, their implementation and use come with challenges, including concerns about data privacy and security, the need for substantial training and adaptation among healthcare professionals, and the potential for increased administrative burden. Addressing these challenges requires ongoing efforts to refine EHR systems, improve user interfaces, and develop policies that protect patient information while maximizing the benefits of digital documentation.

Conclusion

The role of Electronic Health Records in modern healthcare is transformative, offering significant improvements in the efficiency, quality, and safety of patient care. By enhancing the principles of effective documentation and introducing new capabilities, EHRs support a more integrated and patient-centered approach to healthcare delivery. As the healthcare industry continues to evolve, EHRs will remain at the forefront of this change, shaping the future of clinical documentation and healthcare practices.

2.3 Ensuring Patient Privacy and Confidentiality

In the domain of clinical documentation and healthcare delivery, the principles of patient privacy and confidentiality are paramount. These principles are not only ethical imperatives but also legal requirements designed to protect patient information from unauthorized access, use, or disclosure. Ensuring privacy and confidentiality in clinical documentation involves a multifaceted approach that incorporates legal compliance, ethical practice, and the application of technology.

Legal Compliance: HIPAA and Beyond

At the heart of legal compliance in the United States is the Health Insurance Portability and Accountability Act (HIPAA), which sets the standard for the protection of sensitive patient health information. Similar laws exist globally, emphasizing the universal importance of safeguarding patient data. These regulations mandate that healthcare providers and institutions implement appropriate administrative, physical, and technical safeguards to ensure the confidentiality, integrity, and availability of electronic protected health information (ePHI).

Ethical Practice: The Duty to Protect

Beyond legal requirements, healthcare professionals have an ethical duty to maintain patient confidentiality. This duty encompasses respecting the privacy of patient information and discussions, safeguarding against unnecessary disclosure of health data, and ensuring that patient trust is not breached. Ethical practice in documentation requires mindfulness about the information included in patient records and the potential implications of that information being shared.

Technological Safeguards: Encryption and Access Controls

Technological advancements, particularly the adoption of Electronic Health Records (EHRs), offer opportunities to enhance the security of patient information. Encryption technologies ensure that data is unreadable to unauthorized individuals, while access controls limit information access to only those with a legitimate need to know. Audit trails, which record who accessed patient information and when, provide an additional layer of security, enabling the monitoring of compliance with privacy policies and regulations.

Training and Awareness: Building a Culture of Privacy

Ensuring patient privacy and confidentiality extends beyond technology and regulations; it requires cultivating a culture of privacy within healthcare organizations. This involves regular training and awareness programs for all staff members, emphasizing the importance of confidentiality and the proper handling of patient information. Such education ensures that healthcare professionals understand their roles and responsibilities in protecting patient privacy and are equipped to navigate the complexities of information sharing in a healthcare context.

Challenges and Considerations

Despite robust safeguards, challenges persist in ensuring patient privacy and confidentiality. These challenges include the risk of data breaches, the complexities of sharing information for care coordination and telehealth, and the need for clear policies on the de-identification and use of patient data for research. Navigating these challenges requires ongoing vigilance, adaptation to new threats, and a commitment to ethical standards.

Conclusion

The assurance of patient privacy and confidentiality is a cornerstone of trust in the healthcare system. It necessitates a comprehensive approach that integrates legal compliance, ethical practice, technological safeguards, and a culture of privacy. By prioritizing these elements, healthcare providers and institutions can protect sensitive patient information, uphold the principles of medical ethics, and foster a healthcare environment where patients feel secure in sharing their health information.

2.4 Exercise: 10 MCQs with Answers at the End

1. What is the primary purpose of HIPAA in clinical documentation?

   A. To promote the use of electronic health records

   B. To ensure the confidentiality, integrity, and availability of patient information

   C. To standardize medical billing practices

   D. To enhance the quality of healthcare delivery

2. Which principle of effective documentation involves using straightforward language to avoid misunderstandings?

A. Conciseness

B. Clarity

C. Coherence

D. Compliance

3. EHRs improve healthcare delivery by:

A. Reducing the need for patient involvement in their care

B. Limiting access to patient records to a small group of healthcare providers

C. Enhancing communication and access to patient information

D. Decreasing the amount of documentation required

4. Patient portals in EHR systems primarily function to:

A. Enable patients to pay their medical bills online

B. Provide patients access to their own health information

C. Allow patients to write notes in their medical record

D. Give patients the ability to prescribe medications

5. What is a key benefit of standardizing clinical documentation?

A. Reducing the need for patient consent

B. Increasing the complexity of medical records

C. Enhancing the quality of patient care

D. Eliminating the role of healthcare providers in documentation

6. Technological safeguards for patient information include all of the following EXCEPT:

A. Encryption

B. Public Wi-Fi access

C. Access controls

D. Audit trails

7. The ethical duty of healthcare professionals to maintain patient confidentiality is based on:

A. The preference of healthcare institutions

B. The potential for financial gain

C. The trust placed in them by patients

D. The complexity of medical treatments

8. Which is NOT a challenge in ensuring patient privacy and confidentiality?

A. Data breaches

B. Use of encryption technologies

C. Sharing information for care coordination

D. The de-identification of patient data for research

9. A culture of privacy within healthcare organizations is fostered primarily through:

  A. Implementing more advanced technology

  B. Avoiding discussions about privacy and confidentiality

  C. Regular training and awareness programs

  D. Limiting the documentation of sensitive information

10. Coherence in clinical documentation ensures that:

  A. Only the most recent information is included

  B. Information follows a logical flow

  C. Documents are as brief as possible

    D. All healthcare providers use the same documentation software

Answers:

1. B. To ensure the confidentiality, integrity, and availability of patient information

2. B. Clarity

3. C. Enhancing communication and access to patient information

4. B. Provide patients access to their own health information

5. C. Enhancing the quality of patient care

6. B. Public Wi-Fi access

7. C. The trust placed in them by patients

8. B. Use of encryption technologies

9. C. Regular training and awareness programs

10. B. Information follows a logical flow

Chapter 3: Documentation Standards and Regulations

3.1 Overview of Healthcare Regulations

Navigating the landscape of healthcare regulations is a critical aspect of clinical documentation, requiring an understanding of various standards and laws that govern the management, privacy, and security of patient information. These regulations ensure that healthcare delivery is safe, effective, and compliant with national and international guidelines. This overview introduces key healthcare regulations that impact clinical documentation, highlighting their objectives and implications for healthcare providers.

Health Insurance Portability and Accountability Act (HIPAA)

At the forefront of healthcare regulations in the United States is the Health Insurance Portability and Accountability Act (HIPAA), enacted to protect patient privacy and secure sensitive health information. HIPAA sets the standard for handling protected health information (PHI), requiring healthcare providers to implement safeguards to ensure the confidentiality, integrity, and availability of PHI. Compliance with HIPAA is mandatory, and violations can result in significant fines and legal penalties.

The Health Information Technology for Economic and Clinical Health (HITECH) Act

The HITECH Act, a part of the American Recovery and Reinvestment Act of 2009, promotes the adoption and meaningful use of health information technology, particularly electronic health records (EHRs). It strengthens the privacy and security protections established under HIPAA, especially in the context of electronic transmission of health information, and provides incentives for healthcare providers to adopt EHRs.

General Data Protection Regulation (GDPR)

For healthcare organizations operating in or dealing with patients from the European Union, the General Data Protection Regulation (GDPR) imposes strict guidelines on the processing of personal data. GDPR emphasizes the rights of individuals over their personal data, requiring consent for data processing and granting individuals the right to access, correct, and delete their data. GDPR's broad scope and stringent requirements have global implications, affecting healthcare providers worldwide.

The Joint Commission Standards

The Joint Commission, an independent, non-profit organization, accredits and certifies healthcare organizations in the United States. Its standards focus on improving healthcare quality and patient safety, including comprehensive requirements for documentation. Accreditation by The Joint Commission is recognized as a symbol of quality and compliance with the highest performance standards.

Centers for Medicare & Medicaid Services (CMS) Regulations

CMS regulations govern Medicare and Medicaid programs, setting standards for healthcare providers and institutions that receive funding from these programs. These regulations include specific requirements for documentation, billing, and quality of care, aiming to ensure that patients receive medically necessary services and that providers adhere to best practices in healthcare delivery.

Conclusion

Understanding and complying with these and other healthcare regulations is fundamental for healthcare providers. Compliance ensures the protection of patient information, the delivery of high-quality care, and the avoidance of legal and financial penalties. As the healthcare landscape continues to evolve, staying informed about current and emerging regulations will remain a critical responsibility for all involved in clinical documentation and healthcare delivery.

3.2 Navigating Privacy Laws in Healthcare

In the complex field of healthcare, adhering to privacy laws is crucial for protecting patient information and ensuring the confidentiality of health records. These laws, while varying in specific terms and scope across different regions, share common goals: safeguarding personal health information, ensuring patient rights, and setting standards for the secure handling and sharing of this sensitive data. This section delves into navigating these critical regulations without focusing on any single law by name, offering a generalized approach applicable in various jurisdictions.

Understanding the Core Principles

At the heart of these privacy laws are several core principles that healthcare providers must grasp and incorporate into their daily practices. These include the necessity for consent before collecting or sharing patient information, the minimum necessary rule which dictates that only the least amount of information required for a specific purpose should be used or disclosed, and the imperative for implementing both physical and technical safeguards to protect health information against unauthorized access or breaches.

Consent and Patient Rights

Consent is foundational, requiring that patients are informed about how their information will be used and shared and are given the opportunity to agree or object. These laws often grant patients the right to access their health records, request amendments to incorrect or incomplete information, and receive an accounting of disclosures. Healthcare providers must establish clear processes to handle such requests promptly and compliantly.

Implementing Safeguards

To protect patient information, physical, administrative, and technical safeguards are essential. This includes secure storage solutions for physical records, restricted access policies, employee training programs on privacy practices, and the use of encryption and secure transmission protocols for digital data. Conducting regular risk assessments to identify and mitigate potential vulnerabilities is also a key part of maintaining compliance and ensuring the integrity of health information.

Breach Notification

In the event of an unauthorized disclosure of patient information, privacy laws typically require healthcare providers to notify affected individuals and, in some cases, regulatory bodies, within a specific timeframe. Preparing an effective breach response plan is vital, outlining steps to assess the impact, notify stakeholders, and prevent future incidents.

International Considerations

For healthcare providers operating across borders or handling information from international patients, understanding the interplay between local and international privacy laws is crucial. This may involve complying with stricter regulations from other jurisdictions and ensuring seamless adherence to multiple sets of regulations simultaneously.

Conclusion

Navigating the landscape of privacy laws in healthcare is a continuous process, requiring vigilance, ongoing education, and adaptability to legal updates and technological advancements. By grounding their practices in the universal principles of consent, minimum necessary information sharing, robust safeguards, and transparent breach response, healthcare providers can uphold the trust placed in them by patients and the broader community, ensuring the secure and respectful handling of sensitive health information.

3.3 Adhering to International Documentation Standards

In an increasingly globalized world, the healthcare sector is not exempt from the challenges and opportunities presented by international operations and collaborations. Adherence to international documentation standards is crucial for ensuring consistent, high-quality patient care across borders, facilitating research and public health initiatives, and complying with varying legal and regulatory environments. These standards serve as a common language, enabling healthcare providers, researchers, and policymakers to share, compare, and analyze health data effectively and ethically.

The Importance of Standardization

Standardization in clinical documentation ensures that healthcare information is accurate, complete, and accessible, regardless of where the care is provided or the data is analyzed. It supports the interoperability of electronic health record systems, allowing for seamless exchange and utilization of information. This is particularly important for patients receiving care in different countries, for multinational research studies, and for global health monitoring and disease control efforts.

Key International Standards

Several organizations have developed standards to guide clinical documentation practices worldwide. These include:

- **International Classification of Diseases (ICD)**: Developed by the World Health Organization (WHO), the ICD is a globally used diagnostic tool for epidemiology, health management, and clinical purposes. It facilitates the storage and retrieval of diagnostic information and is crucial for billing and health statistics across different countries.

- **Health Level Seven International (HL7)**: HL7 standards provide a framework and related standards for the exchange, integration, sharing, and retrieval of electronic health information. They support clinical practice and the management, delivery, and evaluation of health services.

- **Digital Imaging and Communications in Medicine (DICOM)**: DICOM standards enable the storage, retrieval, processing, and display of medical imaging information, ensuring compatibility and interoperability among different systems used by healthcare professionals.

Implementing International Standards

Adopting international documentation standards involves several steps, including:

- **Training and Education**: Healthcare providers and staff must be trained in the application and implications of these standards to ensure accurate and effective documentation.

- **System Integration**: Electronic health records and other health information systems must be configured or developed to support these standards, ensuring interoperability and compliance.

- **Quality Control and Auditing**: Regular audits and quality control measures are necessary to maintain adherence to international standards, identify areas for improvement, and address any issues promptly.

Challenges and Considerations

While the adoption of international standards offers numerous benefits, it also presents challenges, such as the need for significant investment in technology and training, potential disruptions during the transition period, and the ongoing need to update systems and practices in line with evolving standards. Additionally, healthcare providers must navigate the complexities of integrating these standards within the specific legal and regulatory frameworks of their own countries.

Conclusion

Adhering to international documentation standards is a critical component of modern healthcare, enhancing the quality and continuity of care, facilitating global health initiatives, and supporting the interoperability of health information systems.

By committing to these standards, healthcare providers can better serve their patients, contribute to global health knowledge, and operate effectively in the international healthcare landscape.

3.4 Exercise: 10 MCQs with Answers at the End

1. What is the primary purpose of international documentation standards in healthcare?

   A. To increase healthcare costs

   B. To facilitate global billing processes

   C. To ensure consistent, high-quality patient care across borders

   D. To restrict the sharing of health data

2. Which organization developed the International Classification of Diseases (ICD)?

   A. Health Level Seven International (HL7)

   B. World Health Organization (WHO)

   C. Digital Imaging and Communications in Medicine (DICOM)

   D. Centers for Disease Control and Prevention (CDC)

3. What does HL7 standards primarily facilitate?

A. The exchange of textile manufacturing data

B. The exchange, integration, sharing, and retrieval of electronic health information

C. International travel advisories for healthcare professionals

D. Global pharmaceutical sales data analysis

4. The DICOM standard is specifically designed for:

A. Financial transactions in healthcare

B. Storing, retrieving, processing, and displaying medical imaging information

C. Documenting surgical procedures

D. International drug classification and coding

5. Implementing international documentation standards in healthcare systems requires:

A. Decreased focus on patient care

B. Training and education for healthcare providers

C. Isolation of healthcare systems to prevent data breaches

D. Elimination of electronic health records

6. One of the challenges in adopting international standards is:

   A. The immediate reduction in healthcare delivery costs

   B. The potential need for significant investment in technology and training

   C. The reduction of healthcare quality

   D. Simplification of legal and regulatory compliance

7. Regular audits and quality control measures for documentation standards ensure:

   A. Maintenance of adherence and identification of improvement areas

   B. Decreased healthcare provider accountability

   C. Increased patient wait times for services

   D. Limitation of data sharing between countries

8. The interoperability of electronic health record systems is enhanced by:

   A. Ignoring international standards

   B. Adhering to local documentation practices only

   C. Following international documentation standards

   D. Decreasing the security of health data

9. International documentation standards support global health initiatives by:

   A. Restricting the flow of health information

   B. Allowing for the seamless exchange and utilization of health information

   C. Increasing administrative tasks for healthcare providers

   D. Limiting research and public health monitoring

10. Quality control in the context of international documentation standards refers to:

   A. The restriction of innovative healthcare solutions

   B. Regularly checking adherence to these standards and addressing issues

   C. Decreasing the transparency of healthcare processes

   D. Ignoring updates and evolutions in standards

Answers:

1. C. To ensure consistent, high-quality patient care across borders

2. B. World Health Organization (WHO)

3. B. The exchange, integration, sharing, and retrieval of electronic health information

4. B. Storing, retrieving, processing, and displaying medical imaging information

5. B. Training and education for healthcare providers

6. B. The potential need for significant investment in technology and training

7. A. Maintenance of adherence and identification of improvement areas

8. C. Following international documentation standards

9. B. Allowing for the seamless exchange and utilization of health information

10. B. Regularly checking adherence to these standards and addressing issues

Chapter 4: The Clinical Documentation Improvement Process

4.1 Identifying and Correcting Documentation Gaps

In the realm of healthcare, the integrity of clinical documentation is paramount, not only for ensuring high-quality patient care but also for maintaining compliance with regulatory standards and facilitating accurate billing. Identifying and correcting documentation gaps is a critical component of the Clinical Documentation Improvement (CDI) process, aimed at enhancing the completeness, accuracy, and clarity of medical records.

The Importance of Identifying Documentation Gaps

Documentation gaps can lead to a myriad of issues within the healthcare system, including compromised patient care, regulatory non-compliance, and financial losses. These gaps may arise from incomplete patient records, unclear or ambiguous medical notes, or missing documentation, among other issues. Identifying these gaps is the first step in rectifying inconsistencies and ensuring that the documentation accurately reflects the patient's health status and the care provided.

Strategies for Identifying Documentation Gaps

1. **Regular Audits and Reviews**: Conducting periodic audits of clinical documentation is an effective way to identify patterns of incompleteness or inaccuracies. These audits can be focused on specific departments, types of care, or documentation practices.

2. **Feedback from Healthcare Providers**: Encouraging feedback from physicians, nurses, and other healthcare providers can help identify areas where documentation practices may be lacking or where additional training may be needed.

3. **Analysis of Denials and Rejections**: Reviewing cases of insurance denials and rejections can reveal common documentation issues that prevent accurate billing and reimbursement.

4. **Use of Clinical Documentation Improvement Software**: Leveraging technology, such as CDI software, can automate the process of scanning for documentation gaps, suggesting areas for improvement based on predefined criteria and analytics.

Correcting Documentation Gaps

Once identified, addressing documentation gaps requires a coordinated effort among CDI specialists, healthcare providers, and administrative staff. Strategies include:

1. **Education and Training**: Providing targeted education and training to healthcare providers on best practices in clinical documentation, focusing on areas where gaps have been identified.

2. **Revision and Clarification Processes**: Implementing processes for timely revision and clarification of documentation, including query systems that allow CDI specialists to seek additional information from healthcare providers when gaps or ambiguities are detected.

3. **Enhancing Documentation Templates**: Adjusting electronic health record (EHR) templates and prompts to guide providers in capturing all necessary information can prevent gaps from occurring.

4. **Monitoring and Feedback**: Establishing a system for ongoing monitoring of documentation practices and providing regular feedback to healthcare providers on their documentation quality can promote continuous improvement.

Conclusion

The process of identifying and correcting documentation gaps is a continuous cycle of improvement that is essential for the overall efficacy of the healthcare system. Through diligent efforts in gap identification, targeted education, and process enhancement, healthcare organizations can achieve higher levels of documentation accuracy, thereby improving patient care, compliance, and financial outcomes.

4.2 Strategies for Continuous Improvement

The journey towards excellence in clinical documentation is ongoing, requiring a commitment to continuous improvement. As healthcare environments evolve, so do the standards and expectations for clinical documentation. Strategies for continuous improvement focus on enhancing the accuracy, clarity, and comprehensiveness of medical records, ultimately leading to better patient care, compliance, and operational efficiency. Here are several key strategies that can foster a culture of continuous improvement in clinical documentation.

Implementing a Feedback Loop

A robust feedback loop between clinical documentation specialists, healthcare providers, and coding staff is crucial.

Regularly reviewing documentation practices and outcomes, then providing constructive feedback, helps identify areas for enhancement and acknowledges areas of excellence. This cycle of feedback and improvement encourages learning and development, making it a powerful tool for elevating documentation quality.

Ongoing Education and Training

The landscape of healthcare is constantly changing, with new treatments, technologies, and regulations emerging regularly. Ongoing education and training ensure that all involved in the documentation process are up-to-date on best practices, compliance requirements, and the latest healthcare innovations. Tailored training programs can address specific areas of need, promoting skill development and knowledge expansion across the organization.

Leveraging Technology

Advancements in healthcare technology, including Electronic Health Records (EHRs) and Clinical Documentation Improvement (CDI) software, offer significant opportunities for enhancing documentation practices. These technologies can provide real-time assistance and prompts to healthcare providers, automate the identification of documentation gaps, and facilitate more efficient and accurate documentation processes. Investing in and fully utilizing these technologies can drive significant improvements in documentation quality.

Interdisciplinary Collaboration

Effective clinical documentation improvement requires collaboration across various disciplines within the healthcare setting. Engaging physicians, nurses, allied health professionals, coders, and CDI specialists in a shared mission to enhance documentation can lead to more comprehensive and patient-centered records. Collaborative efforts, such as interdisciplinary rounds or joint documentation review sessions, can foster a deeper understanding of documentation's role in patient care and operational success.

Quality Assurance and Performance Monitoring

Establishing robust quality assurance and performance monitoring processes is essential for tracking improvement over time. This involves setting clear, measurable goals for documentation quality and regularly reviewing performance against these benchmarks. Data-driven approaches allow for the identification of trends, successes, and areas needing attention, guiding strategic efforts to enhance documentation practices.

Promoting a Culture of Quality

Ultimately, the success of continuous improvement strategies depends on cultivating a culture that values quality, accountability, and professional growth. Encouraging open communication, recognizing and rewarding excellence, and creating an environment where feedback is welcomed and acted upon can reinforce the importance of high-quality clinical documentation.

Conclusion

Continuous improvement in clinical documentation is not a goal to be achieved but a process to be embraced. By implementing these strategies, healthcare organizations can ensure that their documentation practices not only meet the current standards but are also poised to adapt to future challenges and opportunities. This commitment to excellence supports the ultimate goal of providing high-quality patient care, maintaining compliance, and enhancing operational efficiency.

4.3 Engaging with Clinicians for Better Documentation

Engaging clinicians in the process of improving clinical documentation is essential for achieving high-quality patient care, accurate billing, and compliance with healthcare regulations. Clinicians, including doctors, nurses, and other healthcare providers, are at the forefront of patient care and play a pivotal role in documenting health information. Their active participation and commitment to documentation excellence can significantly impact the effectiveness of clinical documentation improvement (CDI) initiatives. Here are strategies to foster clinician engagement and promote better documentation practices.

Communication and Collaboration

Open and effective communication is the cornerstone of engaging clinicians in documentation improvement. Regular meetings, interdisciplinary rounds, and feedback sessions can provide opportunities for clinicians to discuss documentation challenges and solutions collaboratively. Creating a platform where clinicians feel heard and their input is valued encourages their active participation in the CDI process.

Education and Training

Tailored education and training sessions that address specific documentation issues relevant to clinicians' daily practices can enhance their understanding and commitment to documentation improvement. Highlighting the impact of accurate documentation on patient care outcomes, regulatory compliance, and financial reimbursement can underscore the importance of their role in the documentation process.

Incorporating Clinician Feedback

Involving clinicians in the development and refinement of documentation processes, including the design of templates and workflows in electronic health record (EHR) systems, ensures that these tools align with their needs and preferences. Actively seeking and incorporating clinician feedback can lead to more user-friendly documentation practices that enhance efficiency and accuracy.

Providing Support and Resources

Offering dedicated support, such as CDI specialists or documentation coaches, can assist clinicians with real-time documentation challenges. These resources can offer immediate guidance, clarification, and support, minimizing the burden on clinicians and allowing them to focus on patient care while maintaining documentation standards.

Recognizing and Rewarding Excellence

Recognizing and rewarding clinicians who consistently demonstrate excellence in documentation can motivate others to improve their documentation practices. Recognition programs, awards, or acknowledgments in staff meetings can highlight the value placed on high-quality documentation and encourage a culture of excellence.

Demonstrating the Impact of Quality Documentation

Sharing success stories and data that illustrate the positive impact of improved documentation on patient care outcomes, financial performance, and compliance can motivate clinicians to prioritize documentation. Seeing tangible results of their efforts can reinforce the importance of their contributions to the organization's goals.

Simplifying Documentation Processes

Streamlining documentation processes and reducing administrative burdens can enhance clinician engagement. Simplifying templates, minimizing redundant data entry, and optimizing EHR functionalities can make documentation more efficient and less time-consuming, allowing clinicians to allocate more time to patient care.

Conclusion

Engaging clinicians in the process of improving clinical documentation requires a multifaceted approach that emphasizes communication, collaboration, and support. By aligning documentation practices with clinicians' workflows, providing education and resources, and recognizing their efforts, healthcare organizations can foster a culture of documentation excellence that supports high-quality patient care, regulatory compliance, and operational efficiency.

4.4 Exercise: 10 MCQs with Answers at the End

Let's design a set of 10 multiple-choice questions (MCQs) based on the themes covered in Chapter 4, focusing on the clinical documentation improvement process, strategies for continuous improvement, engaging with clinicians, and identifying and correcting documentation gaps. This exercise aims to reinforce key concepts and assess understanding.

1. What is the primary goal of the Clinical Documentation Improvement (CDI) process?

  A) Reducing the time clinicians spend on documentation

  B) Improving the quality and accuracy of patient records

  C) Increasing the hospital's revenue

  D) Simplifying medical terminology

2. Regular audits and reviews of clinical documentation help identify:

  A) The most efficient documentation software

  B) Patterns of incompleteness or inaccuracies

  C) The best-performing departments

  D) Opportunities for reducing staff

3. Which strategy is NOT effective for correcting documentation gaps?

  A) Penalizing clinicians for errors

  B) Providing targeted education and training

  C) Implementing revision and clarification processes

  D) Enhancing documentation templates

4. Engaging clinicians in documentation improvement is crucial because:

A) They are responsible for entering billing codes

B) They play a pivotal role in documenting health information

C) They prefer using paper-based records

D) They have a lot of free time

5. Tailored education and training sessions for clinicians should NOT:

A) Focus solely on the financial aspects of documentation

B) Address specific documentation issues relevant to their practices

C) Highlight the impact of accurate documentation on patient care

D) Be based on feedback and identified documentation gaps

6. The use of Clinical Documentation Improvement (CDI) software is primarily to:

A) Replace the need for clinician documentation

B) Automate the process of scanning for documentation gaps

C) Eliminate the need for audits and reviews

D) Train new staff members

7. Effective communication and collaboration in CDI processes include:

A) Ignoring clinician feedback

B) Regular meetings and feedback sessions

C) Limiting information sharing between departments

D) Using medical jargon as much as possible

8. Which is NOT a benefit of engaging clinicians in improving documentation?

A) Enhanced patient care

B) Increased administrative workload for clinicians

C) Improved accuracy of patient records

D) Better compliance with healthcare regulations

9. A feedback loop in the CDI process is important because it:

A) Allows for punitive actions against underperforming clinicians

B) Enables continuous learning and development

C) Is only necessary for legal compliance

D) Reduces the need for technology in documentation

10. Simplifying documentation processes can lead to:

A) Less time allocated to patient care

B) Greater clinician engagement and efficiency

C) Decreased accuracy in patient records

D) More complex workflows

Answers:

1. B) Improving the quality and accuracy of patient records

2. B) Patterns of incompleteness or inaccuracies

3. A) Penalizing clinicians for errors

4. B) They play a pivotal role in documenting health information

5. A) Focus solely on the financial aspects of documentation

6. B) Automate the process of scanning for documentation gaps

7. B) Regular meetings and feedback sessions

8. B) Increased administrative workload for clinicians

9. B) Enables continuous learning and development

10. B) Greater clinician engagement and efficiency

Chapter 5: Risk Management in Clinical Documentation

5.1 Mitigating Legal Risks Through Documentation

In the complex landscape of healthcare, legal risks loom large, particularly in areas related to patient care and clinical documentation. Properly managed, clinical documentation can serve as a robust tool for mitigating these risks, safeguarding both patients and healthcare providers against potential legal complications. This section explores strategies for utilizing clinical documentation to minimize legal vulnerabilities and enhance overall patient safety.

The Role of Documentation in Legal Protection

Clinical documentation serves several critical functions in the legal arena: it provides a detailed record of patient care, supports decision-making processes, and demonstrates compliance with applicable standards and regulations. In litigation or audits, comprehensive and accurate documentation can substantiate the quality and appropriateness of care provided, serving as evidence that healthcare providers acted competently and in line with best practices.

Strategies for Mitigating Legal Risks

1. **Ensure Comprehensive and Accurate Records**: Every patient interaction, treatment decision, and care outcome should be thoroughly documented in the patient's medical record. This includes noting informed consent, patient education, and any deviations from standard protocols, along with the rationale for such decisions.

2. **Adherence to Standards of Care**: Documentation should reflect adherence to accepted standards of care and guidelines. This not only supports the delivery of high-quality healthcare but also provides a defense against claims of negligence or substandard care.

3. **Timely Documentation**: Entries should be made as close to the time of the patient encounter as possible to ensure accuracy and completeness. Delayed documentation is less reliable and more susceptible to challenges in legal proceedings.

4. **Clarity and Objectivity**: Documentation should be clear, objective, and free of ambiguous language. Subjective opinions or derogatory comments have no place in clinical records and can undermine the professionalism and credibility of the documentation in a legal context.

5. **Documentation of Patient Communication**: Detailed records of discussions with patients about their condition, treatment options, potential risks, and expected outcomes are essential.

This demonstrates that patients were informed and involved in their care decisions, which is crucial in defending against claims of inadequate consent or patient education.

6. **Regular Training and Education**: Healthcare providers should receive ongoing training in documentation practices, legal aspects of healthcare, and risk management. This ensures that all staff are aware of the importance of documentation in legal protection and are equipped with the skills to document effectively.

7. **Use of Electronic Health Records (EHRs)**: EHRs offer functionalities that can enhance the accuracy and efficiency of documentation, such as time-stamped entries, audit trails, and templates that prompt for complete information. Leveraging these tools can further mitigate legal risks.

Conclusion

Mitigating legal risks through effective clinical documentation is an essential aspect of healthcare risk management. By ensuring that documentation is comprehensive, accurate, timely, and adherent to standards of care, healthcare providers can protect themselves and their patients from the potential adverse effects of legal challenges. Incorporating best practices in documentation into daily routines not only enhances patient care but also fortifies the legal and professional standing of healthcare providers.

5.2 Handling Documentation Errors

In the complex and fast-paced environment of healthcare, documentation errors are not uncommon, yet they can have significant implications for patient care, legal compliance, and the reputation of healthcare providers. Handling these errors appropriately is crucial for maintaining the integrity of the medical record, ensuring patient safety, and mitigating potential legal and regulatory risks. This section outlines effective strategies for managing documentation errors, emphasizing the importance of transparency, accuracy, and ethical practices.

Identification and Acknowledgment

The first step in handling documentation errors is timely identification. This can be facilitated by regular audits, peer reviews, and the use of electronic health record (EHR) systems that flag inconsistencies or irregularities. Once an error is identified, it must be acknowledged openly. The culture within healthcare organizations should encourage the reporting of errors without fear of punitive measures, fostering an environment of continuous improvement and learning.

Correcting Errors

When correcting documentation errors, the following practices are paramount:

- **Do Not Erase or Obscure the Original Entry**: Altering the original content can lead to suspicions of tampering and can compromise the integrity of the medical record. In paper records, errors should be crossed out with a single line, ensuring the original text is still legible. In electronic records, utilize the system's functionality for making corrections, which typically includes an audit trail that records the original entry and the correction.

- **Make a New Entry**: Clearly indicate that this entry corrects a previous error. Include the date, time, and rationale for the correction, and reference the original erroneous entry if possible. This new entry should be made as soon as the error is discovered to maintain the chronological accuracy of the record.

- **Be Transparent and Objective**: The correction should objectively describe the error and the correction without placing blame or making subjective comments. This transparency maintains the trustworthiness of the medical record.

Training and Education

Ongoing education and training on proper documentation practices are crucial for preventing errors. Training programs should cover the ethical and legal implications of accurate documentation, how to identify and correct errors, and the importance of an honest and transparent approach to error correction.

Implementing Systematic Changes

Analyzing documentation errors can provide valuable insights into systemic issues that may contribute to these mistakes. Healthcare organizations should use this information to implement changes in processes, training, or EHR systems to prevent future errors. This might include adjusting templates, improving user interfaces, or introducing additional checks and balances in the documentation process.

Legal and Ethical Considerations

Handling documentation errors with integrity is not only a matter of best practice but also a legal and ethical obligation. Corrections should be made in a way that preserves the integrity of the medical record and upholds the principles of patient care and confidentiality. In cases where an error has the potential to harm a patient, it is essential to inform the patient and take appropriate steps to address any adverse effects.

Conclusion

Effectively managing documentation errors is a critical component of risk management in healthcare. By fostering a culture that prioritizes accuracy, transparency, and ethical practices, healthcare organizations can mitigate the risks associated with documentation errors, enhance patient safety, and maintain the trust of patients and the wider healthcare community.

5.3 Documentation Audits: Purpose and Process

Documentation audits play a pivotal role in the healthcare quality improvement process, serving as a systematic review of clinical records to ensure accuracy, completeness, and compliance with established standards and regulations. These audits are instrumental in identifying discrepancies, areas for improvement, and best practices, ultimately leading to enhanced patient care, legal compliance, and organizational efficiency. Understanding the purpose and process of documentation audits is essential for healthcare providers and administrators alike.

Purpose of Documentation Audits

- **Compliance Assurance**: Audits verify adherence to legal, regulatory, and accreditation standards, helping to avoid penalties and ensuring patient rights are protected.

- **Quality Improvement**: By identifying gaps and inconsistencies in documentation, audits provide insights into areas needing improvement, contributing to better patient outcomes and care continuity.

- **Risk Management**: Audits help mitigate legal and financial risks by ensuring documentation accurately reflects the care provided, supporting billing and reimbursement processes.

- **Educational Opportunities**: Findings from audits can highlight areas where additional training or resources are needed, guiding educational efforts to enhance staff competencies.

Audit Process

1. Planning and Preparation

- **Define Objectives**: Clearly outline what the audit aims to achieve, whether it's assessing compliance with a specific regulation, improving clinical outcomes, or evaluating coding accuracy.

- **Select Samples**: Choose a representative sample of records to audit. This may be random or targeted based on prior issues or high-risk areas.

- **Develop Audit Tools and Criteria**: Utilize checklists, scoring systems, and guidelines that reflect current standards and best practices to evaluate documentation.

2. Conducting the Audit

- **Review Selected Records**: Examine the documentation within each selected record according to the predefined criteria. Pay attention to detail and maintain objectivity.

- **Collect Data**: Gather findings from the review process, noting areas of non-compliance, exemplary documentation, and potential areas for improvement.

3. Analysis and Reporting

- **Analyze Findings**: Evaluate the data to identify trends, common errors, and areas of strength. Compare results against benchmarks or goals.

- **Prepare a Report**: Summarize the audit findings, including areas of compliance, discrepancies, and recommendations for improvement.

4. Post-Audit Actions

- **Feedback and Education**: Share the audit results with relevant staff and stakeholders. Provide constructive feedback and, if necessary, organize training sessions to address identified gaps.

- **Implement Improvements**: Based on audit findings, make necessary changes to policies, procedures, or documentation practices. This may involve updating templates, enhancing EHR functionalities, or revising workflows.

- **Monitor Progress**: After implementing changes, continue to monitor documentation practices to assess the effectiveness of interventions and ensure sustained improvements.

5. Continuous Improvement

- Establish a schedule for regular documentation audits as part of an ongoing quality improvement process. Continuous auditing allows for the timely identification and correction of issues, fostering a culture of excellence and accountability in clinical documentation.

Conclusion

Documentation audits are a critical component of effective healthcare management, offering a structured approach to evaluating and enhancing the quality of clinical documentation. By systematically reviewing and analyzing clinical records, healthcare organizations can ensure compliance, improve patient care, and reduce risk, thereby achieving their overarching goal of delivering high-quality healthcare services.

5.4 Exercise: 10 MCQs with Answers at the End

1. What is the primary goal of conducting documentation audits in healthcare?

   A) To penalize healthcare providers

   B) To improve patient care through accurate documentation

   C) To reduce the workload of healthcare staff

   D) To increase the healthcare facility's revenue

2. Which of the following is NOT a purpose of documentation audits?

   A) Assuring compliance with legal standards

   B) Identifying educational opportunities for staff

C) Guaranteeing patient satisfaction with healthcare services

D) Managing risks associated with documentation errors

3. When correcting documentation errors, it is important to:

A) Erase the error completely to maintain document neatness

B) Make corrections in a way that the original error is still legible

C) Avoid documenting the correction to prevent legal issues

D) Correct errors anonymously to avoid accountability

4. Effective handling of documentation errors includes:

A) Punishing staff who make errors to deter future mistakes

B) Using errors as learning opportunities to improve practices

C) Ignoring minor errors as they have minimal impact

D) Covering up errors to protect the facility's reputation

5. What is an essential step in the process of conducting a documentation audit?

A) Selecting a sample of records at random without specific criteria

B) Defining clear objectives for what the audit aims to achieve

C) Focusing solely on the negative aspects of documentation

D) Conducting audits without informing the healthcare staff involved

6. How should findings from documentation audits be used?

   A) To single out and discipline underperforming staff

   B) As a basis for continuous improvement and staff training

   C) Solely for reporting to external regulatory bodies

   D) To justify budget cuts in healthcare services

7. In the context of documentation audits, what does 'compliance assurance' refer to?

   A) Ensuring all staff comply with management's directives

   B) Verifying adherence to internal policies only

   C) Confirming documentation meets legal, regulatory, and accreditation standards

   D) Guaranteeing that all patient feedback is positive

8. Which strategy is not recommended for engaging clinicians in documentation improvement?

   A) Offering incentives for the best-documented cases

   B) Ignoring their feedback and suggestions

   C) Providing targeted education and resources

   D) Involving them in the development of documentation tools

9. A culture that encourages reporting and correcting documentation errors without fear of punitive measures can lead to:

  A) Decreased staff morale and performance

  B) Increased errors due to lack of consequences

  C) An environment of continuous improvement and learning

  D) A disregard for documentation standards

10. Regular documentation audits are essential because they:

  A) Create additional paperwork and processes

  B) Help maintain high standards of patient care and compliance

  C) Are a formality that healthcare facilities must endure

  D) Discourage staff from making any documentation at all

Answers:

1. B) To improve patient care through accurate documentation

2. C) Guaranteeing patient satisfaction with healthcare services

3. B) Make corrections in a way that the original error is still legible

4. B) Using errors as learning opportunities to improve practices

5. B) Defining clear objectives for what the audit aims to achieve

6. B) As a basis for continuous improvement and staff training

7. C) Confirming documentation meets legal, regulatory, and accreditation standards

8. B) Ignoring their feedback and suggestions

9. C) An environment of continuous improvement and learning

10. B) Help maintain high standards of patient care and compliance

Chapter 6: Specialty-Specific Documentation Challenges

6.1 Documentation in Surgical Practices

Documentation in surgical practices presents unique challenges and requirements that are critical for ensuring patient safety, effective communication among healthcare providers, and compliance with regulatory and billing requirements. Surgical documentation encompasses a wide range of data, from pre-operative assessments to post-operative care and follow-up. Addressing the specific challenges of surgical documentation is essential for maintaining high standards of patient care and operational efficiency in these settings.

Pre-operative Documentation

The pre-operative phase involves detailed documentation of patient assessments, including medical history, physical examinations, and the results of diagnostic tests. Documenting informed consent is crucial in this phase, requiring clear communication with the patient about the risks, benefits, and alternatives to the proposed surgical procedure. This documentation must be thorough and accurate, providing a solid foundation for surgical planning and patient education.

Intra-operative Documentation

Intra-operative documentation captures the critical details of the surgical procedure itself. This includes the surgical team members, the time the surgery started and ended, the types of anesthesia used, a detailed account of the surgical procedure, any complications encountered, and the condition of the patient at the end of the surgery. The surgical narrative must be precise and comprehensive, ensuring that any healthcare provider reviewing the record can understand exactly what occurred during the procedure.

Post-operative Documentation

Post-operative documentation focuses on the patient's recovery and includes notes on the immediate post-operative care, the patient's response to the surgery, any complications, pain management, and instructions given to the patient upon discharge. This phase of documentation is vital for coordinating ongoing care and evaluating the outcome of the surgical intervention.

Challenges in Surgical Documentation

- **Complexity and Detail**: The intricate details of surgical procedures require precise and comprehensive documentation, which can be time-consuming and complex.

- **Dynamic Surgical Environment**: The fast-paced and unpredictable nature of surgical environments can make real-time documentation challenging.

- **Compliance and Billing**: Accurate documentation is essential for compliance with healthcare regulations and for billing purposes. Surgical documentation must meet specific criteria to support reimbursement claims, requiring an in-depth understanding of coding and billing practices.

- **Interdisciplinary Communication**: Effective surgical documentation must facilitate communication among a wide range of professionals, including surgeons, anesthesiologists, nurses, and post-operative care providers. Ensuring consistency and clarity across diverse teams is a significant challenge.

Strategies for Improving Surgical Documentation

- **Standardization of Forms and Checklists**: Using standardized documentation forms and surgical checklists can help ensure that all critical information is captured consistently and thoroughly.

- **Education and Training**: Ongoing education and training for surgical staff on documentation practices, regulatory requirements, and the use of electronic health record systems can improve the accuracy and efficiency of documentation.

- **Technology Integration**: Leveraging technology, such as voice recognition software for dictation or integrated EHR systems, can streamline the documentation process and reduce the burden on surgical staff.

- **Collaborative Review Processes**: Implementing collaborative review and feedback processes for surgical documentation can help identify areas for improvement and ensure that documentation meets the required standards for patient care and compliance.

Conclusion

Documentation in surgical practices involves navigating a range of challenges, from the complexity of capturing detailed surgical procedures to ensuring compliance with regulatory requirements. By adopting strategic approaches to documentation, surgical teams can enhance patient safety, improve communication among healthcare providers, and meet the demands of an increasingly complex healthcare environment.

6.2 Managing Records in Pediatric Care

Pediatric care presents unique challenges and considerations in clinical documentation, stemming from the ongoing growth and development of patients, the involvement of family members in care decisions, and the need for a child-centric approach to healthcare. Effective management of pediatric records requires attention to detail, an understanding of developmental milestones, and a collaborative approach to healthcare delivery.

Unique Aspects of Pediatric Documentation

- **Developmental Milestones**: Documentation in pediatric care must include detailed records of a child's physical, emotional, and cognitive development. Tracking and recording developmental milestones are crucial for identifying potential developmental delays or concerns early on.

- **Immunization Records**: Pediatric records must meticulously document immunizations, ensuring that children receive vaccinations according to recommended schedules and that any adverse reactions are promptly recorded.

- **Family and Social History**: Given the impact of family and social environments on a child's health, pediatric documentation should include comprehensive information on family health history, living conditions, and any social issues that may affect the child's well-being.

- **Consent and Assent**: Documentation must reflect not only the legal guardians' informed consent for treatments and procedures but also, where appropriate, the assent of older children and adolescents, acknowledging their role in the healthcare decision-making process.

Challenges in Pediatric Documentation

- **Communicating with Children and Families**: Effective pediatric care requires clear communication tailored to the age and understanding of the child, as well as to the concerns and expectations of their families. Documentation must capture these interactions accurately, reflecting shared decision-making processes.

- **Longitudinal Record Keeping**: Pediatric records span the significant portion of a child's development from birth to adulthood. Ensuring continuity and coherence in documentation over many years poses a logistical challenge, requiring efficient systems for managing and updating records.

- **Confidentiality and Privacy**: Especially with adolescent patients, balancing the need for confidentiality with parental rights to access their child's health information requires careful consideration and documentation. Guidelines and laws regarding minors' consent and confidentiality must be meticulously adhered to and reflected in the records.

Strategies for Effective Pediatric Record Management

- **Standardized Growth Charts and Developmental Screening Tools**: Utilizing standardized tools for tracking growth and development helps in the early identification of potential issues and ensures that documentation is consistent and comparable over time.

- **Electronic Health Records (EHRs)**: Implementing EHR systems that are designed with pediatric needs in mind can facilitate the management of developmental data, immunization records, and longitudinal tracking of health information.

- **Education and Training**: Providing ongoing education for healthcare providers on pediatric-specific documentation practices, legal requirements, and effective communication strategies can enhance the quality of pediatric records.

- **Family Engagement**: Involving families in the documentation process, through tools like patient portals, can improve the accuracy of health histories, ensure adherence to treatment plans, and enhance the overall quality of pediatric care.

Conclusion

Managing records in pediatric care requires an approach that is sensitive to the unique needs and challenges of treating children. By focusing on developmental milestones, ensuring accurate immunization records, and fostering effective communication with families, healthcare providers can maintain comprehensive and meaningful pediatric records. Embracing technology and ongoing education are key to navigating the complexities of pediatric documentation, ultimately contributing to better health outcomes and a more collaborative approach to child health care.

6.3 Behavioral Health Documentation Nuances

Behavioral health documentation involves unique challenges and considerations, reflecting the complexity of diagnosing and treating mental health and substance use disorders. The sensitive nature of behavioral health information demands a nuanced approach to documentation, prioritizing patient confidentiality, therapeutic relationships, and the accurate representation of clinical encounters. Understanding these nuances is essential for providing effective care and supporting the recovery process.

Key Considerations in Behavioral Health Documentation

- **Patient Confidentiality**: Given the stigma often associated with mental health issues, maintaining patient confidentiality is paramount. Documentation should be accessible only to individuals directly involved in the patient's care, with strict adherence to privacy laws and regulations.

- **Therapeutic Alliance**: The notes should respect the therapeutic alliance between the patient and the provider. Documentation practices should not interfere with the development of trust, and the language used should be neutral, avoiding judgment or bias.

- **Holistic and Person-Centered Care**: Behavioral health documentation should reflect a holistic view of the patient, considering not only symptoms and treatment but also the patient's strengths, preferences, and goals. This approach supports person-centered care, emphasizing the patient's active role in their recovery journey.

Challenges in Behavioral Health Documentation

- **Subjectivity and Complexity**: Documenting mental health conditions can be inherently more subjective than other medical fields, requiring careful attention to language to accurately convey the patient's status and the clinician's assessment.

- **Legal and Ethical Considerations**: Behavioral health professionals must navigate complex legal and ethical landscapes, balancing the need for documentation with the patient's right to privacy. This includes considerations around duty to warn, involuntary commitment, and minors' rights.

- **Continuity and Coordination of Care**: Accurate and comprehensive documentation is crucial for facilitating continuity and coordination of care, especially for patients receiving services from multiple providers or transitioning between levels of care.

Strategies for Effective Behavioral Health Documentation

- **Use of Standardized Assessment Tools**: Incorporating standardized scales and assessments can help objectify and clarify clinical findings, making it easier to track progress over time and communicate with other providers.

- **Training and Sensitivity**: Ongoing training in culturally sensitive, trauma-informed care and documentation practices can help providers approach documentation in a manner that respects and empowers patients.

- **Leveraging Technology**: Electronic health records (EHRs) and other digital tools can enhance the efficiency and quality of documentation, providing templates and prompts to ensure completeness while facilitating secure sharing of information with authorized team members.

- **Collaboration and Consent**: Engaging patients in the documentation process, including discussing how information will be used and obtaining informed consent for the release of information, can enhance trust and cooperation.

Conclusion

Behavioral health documentation requires careful consideration of various nuances to ensure it serves its intended purpose without compromising patient care or confidentiality. By adopting a person-centered, ethical, and legally compliant approach to documentation, behavioral health providers can support effective treatment planning, continuity of care, and the therapeutic relationship, ultimately contributing to better patient outcomes.

6.4 Exercise: 10 MCQs with Answers at the End

1. What is a primary consideration in behavioral health documentation?

   A) Maximizing the use of medical jargon

   B) Prioritizing patient confidentiality

   C) Focusing solely on negative patient behaviors

   D) Ignoring legal and ethical standards

2. Effective behavioral health documentation should:

   A) Exclude the patient's strengths and preferences

   B) Be accessible to anyone interested in the patient's care

C) Reflect a holistic view of the patient

D) Avoid documenting treatment goals and progress

3. A key challenge in behavioral health documentation is:

A) The straightforward nature of the data

B) Maintaining a judgmental tone to motivate patients

C) Balancing subjectivity with accurate clinical assessments

D) Reducing the amount of documentation to save time

4. Standardized assessment tools in behavioral health are used to:

A) Decrease the reliability of diagnoses

B) Objectify and clarify clinical findings

C) Complicate the treatment process

D) Discourage patient involvement in care

5. Legal and ethical considerations in behavioral health documentation include all except:

A) Patient's right to privacy

B) Duty to warn in situations of imminent harm

C) Universal access to patient records

D) Involuntary commitment procedures

6. The therapeutic alliance is:

A) Negatively impacted by accurate documentation

B) Irrelevant to documentation practices

C) Supported by neutral and nonjudgmental language

D) Strengthened by withholding information from the patient

7. Continuity and coordination of care in behavioral health are facilitated by:

A) Limiting documentation to minimize paperwork

B) Accurate and comprehensive documentation

C) Keeping records private from other healthcare providers

D) Using vague descriptions to maintain confidentiality

8. Training in behavioral health documentation should emphasize:

A) The exclusive use of positive patient descriptors

B) Culturally sensitive and trauma-informed practices

C) Avoidance of documenting legal and ethical considerations

D) Reducing the frequency of documentation updates

9. The use of Electronic Health Records (EHRs) in behavioral health documentation helps to:

A) Decrease the security of patient information

B) Ensure completeness and facilitate secure sharing of information

C) Eliminate the need for patient consent in documentation

D) Discourage collaboration among healthcare providers

10. A person-centered approach in behavioral health documentation:

A) Excludes the patient's goals and preferences

B) Focuses only on medical treatment without considering holistic care

C) Prioritizes the patient's strengths, preferences, and goals

D) Assumes that the provider knows best, minimizing patient input

Answers:

1. B) Prioritizing patient confidentiality

2. C) Reflect a holistic view of the patient

3. C) Balancing subjectivity with accurate clinical assessments

4. B) Objectify and clarify clinical findings

5. C) Universal access to patient records

6. C) Supported by neutral and nonjudgmental language

7. B) Accurate and comprehensive documentation

8. B) Culturally sensitive and trauma-informed practices

9. B) Ensure completeness and facilitate secure sharing of information

10. C) Prioritizes the patient's strengths, preferences, and goals

Chapter 7: Technology and Clinical Documentation

7.1 Leveraging EHRs for Improved Documentation

Electronic Health Records (EHRs) have transformed the landscape of clinical documentation, offering unparalleled opportunities for enhancing the quality, efficiency, and accessibility of patient records. By leveraging EHRs, healthcare providers can improve documentation practices, facilitate better patient care, and meet regulatory compliance more effectively. This section explores how EHRs can be utilized to their fullest potential in clinical documentation.

Enhanced Accessibility and Coordination

EHRs centralize patient data, making it accessible to authorized healthcare providers across different locations and specialties. This accessibility improves coordination of care, as providers can easily share and review patient information, reducing the risk of errors and duplicative tests. By having a comprehensive view of a patient's health history, providers can make informed decisions, leading to better patient outcomes.

Standardization and Compliance

EHR systems often come with built-in templates and standardized forms that guide healthcare providers in capturing all necessary information. This standardization not only ensures completeness but also aids in compliance with healthcare regulations. Templates can be customized to meet the specific documentation requirements of different specialties, ensuring that records are consistent and adhere to best practices.

Real-time Documentation and Alerts

One of the key advantages of EHRs is the ability to document care in real-time. This immediacy ensures that patient records are up-to-date and reflects the most current information. Additionally, EHRs can provide alerts and reminders for preventative care measures, follow-ups, and medication management, enhancing the quality of care and patient safety.

Data Analytics and Quality Improvement

EHRs are invaluable tools for data analytics, offering insights into patient outcomes, practice patterns, and areas for improvement. By analyzing data from EHRs, healthcare organizations can identify trends, track performance against quality metrics, and implement evidence-based practices. This analytical capability supports continuous quality improvement and contributes to the advancement of healthcare delivery.

Patient Engagement and Empowerment

Modern EHR systems often include patient portals that enable patients to access their health records, view lab results, request appointments, and communicate with their healthcare providers. This engagement empowers patients to take an active role in their healthcare, improving adherence to treatment plans and patient satisfaction.

Overcoming Challenges

While EHRs offer numerous benefits, challenges such as user interface complexity, data entry burden, and interoperability issues can hinder their effectiveness. Addressing these challenges requires ongoing training, user-centered design improvements, and the adoption of standards for data exchange. Collaboration among healthcare providers, EHR vendors, and regulatory bodies is essential to optimize the use of EHRs in clinical documentation.

Conclusion

Leveraging EHRs for improved documentation represents a significant step forward in the evolution of healthcare delivery. By enhancing accessibility, standardization, real-time documentation, data analytics, and patient engagement, EHRs play a critical role in advancing patient care, safety, and satisfaction. Overcoming the challenges associated with EHR implementation and use is vital for realizing the full potential of this technology in clinical documentation.

7.2 The Impact of AI and Machine Learning

The advent of Artificial Intelligence (AI) and Machine Learning (ML) in healthcare has ushered in a new era of innovation, particularly in the realm of clinical documentation. These technologies offer the potential to significantly enhance the efficiency, accuracy, and quality of patient records, ultimately improving patient care and healthcare outcomes. Here, we delve into the transformative impact of AI and ML on clinical documentation.

Automated Documentation and Data Entry

AI-powered tools can automate the tedious and time-consuming task of data entry, reducing the administrative burden on healthcare providers. Natural Language Processing (NLP) algorithms can interpret free-text notes, extract relevant information, and populate structured fields in Electronic Health Records (EHRs), ensuring that patient records are comprehensive and up-to-date.

Enhanced Accuracy and Consistency

Machine Learning algorithms can analyze vast amounts of data to identify patterns, anomalies, and trends. In the context of clinical documentation, this capability can be harnessed to flag inconsistencies, potential errors, or omissions in patient records, prompting healthcare providers to review and correct the information. This leads to more accurate and consistent documentation, enhancing patient safety and care quality.

Predictive Analytics for Improved Patient Care

AI and ML can analyze historical and real-time patient data to predict health outcomes, enabling proactive management of patient care. For instance, predictive analytics can identify patients at high risk for readmission, allowing healthcare teams to implement targeted interventions. This predictive capability extends to suggesting personalized treatment plans based on the analysis of similar patient profiles and outcomes, thereby improving the effectiveness of care.

Voice Recognition and Transcription

Voice recognition technology, powered by AI, allows healthcare providers to dictate clinical notes verbally, which are then accurately transcribed and integrated into the EHR. This technology streamlines documentation processes, reduces manual data entry errors, and allows providers to focus more on patient interaction rather than paperwork.

Interoperability and Data Integration

AI and ML play a crucial role in improving the interoperability of healthcare systems, facilitating seamless data exchange between different EHR systems and healthcare providers. By standardizing data formats and employing intelligent algorithms to interpret and integrate data, these technologies ensure that patient records are complete, accurate, and accessible across the care continuum.

Challenges and Ethical Considerations

While AI and ML offer significant benefits, their implementation in clinical documentation is not without challenges. Issues such as data privacy, security, and the need for transparent algorithms that can be audited and explained are paramount. Additionally, there is a need for ongoing training and adaptation among healthcare providers to effectively integrate these technologies into clinical practice.

Conclusion

The impact of AI and Machine Learning on clinical documentation is profound, offering opportunities to enhance the efficiency, accuracy, and quality of patient records. As these technologies continue to evolve and integrate into healthcare systems, they promise to transform the landscape of clinical documentation, supporting better patient outcomes and the advancement of healthcare delivery. However, navigating the challenges and ethical considerations associated with AI and ML will be crucial for realizing their full potential in improving clinical documentation.

7.3 Telehealth Documentation Considerations

The rise of telehealth as a mode of delivering healthcare services has introduced new considerations for clinical documentation. Telehealth, which encompasses a broad range of technologies to deliver virtual medical, health, and education services, has become increasingly important, especially in response to global health challenges and the need for accessible healthcare. The unique aspects of telehealth interactions require adaptations in documentation practices to ensure the quality and continuity of care are maintained. This section explores key considerations for documenting telehealth encounters effectively.

Documenting the Modality of Care

One of the first considerations in telehealth documentation is to clearly indicate that the encounter was conducted via telehealth. This includes specifying the technology used (e.g., video conferencing, telephone call, secure messaging) and any relevant details about the virtual setting. Documenting the modality of care is important for billing purposes, regulatory compliance, and clarifying the context of the healthcare interaction.

Consent for Virtual Visits

Documenting patient consent for telehealth services is crucial. Consent should cover the use of technology for healthcare delivery, including an acknowledgment of its limitations and the security measures in place to protect patient privacy. This consent can be verbal or written, depending on jurisdictional requirements, but must be clearly documented in the patient's record.

Technical and Environmental Factors

The quality of telehealth services can be influenced by technical and environmental factors, such as internet connectivity, the quality of audio/video, and the privacy of the location from which the patient is participating. Documenting these factors can provide context for the encounter, especially if technical issues impact the quality of the consultation or the accuracy of assessments made during the visit.

Clinical Observations and Limitations

During telehealth encounters, certain clinical observations may be limited by the virtual format. For example, physical examinations are restricted compared to in-person visits. It's important to document these limitations, including any aspects of the assessment that could not be fully evaluated through telehealth. This information is vital for future care decisions and understanding the scope of the telehealth consultation.

Follow-up and Care Coordination

Telehealth documentation should include clear instructions for follow-up care, referrals, and any necessary in-person evaluations. Given the remote nature of telehealth, ensuring continuity of care through precise documentation of recommended next steps is essential. This helps bridge any gaps between virtual and in-person care modalities.

Privacy and Security Measures

Given the use of digital platforms for telehealth, documenting the privacy and security measures in place to protect patient information during the encounter is important. This might include the use of encrypted communication channels, secure patient identification processes, and adherence to privacy regulations specific to telehealth.

Conclusion

Telehealth documentation presents unique challenges and considerations that reflect the virtual nature of these healthcare encounters. By meticulously documenting the modality of care, patient consent, technical and environmental factors, clinical observations, follow-up care, and privacy measures, healthcare providers can ensure that telehealth services are delivered with the same level of quality, accountability, and continuity as traditional in-person care. As telehealth continues to evolve, so too will the standards and practices for its documentation, necessitating ongoing adaptation and education for healthcare providers.

7.4 Exercise: 10 MCQs with Answers at the End

1. What is essential to document at the beginning of a telehealth visit?

   A) The physical location of the provider

   B) The modality of the telehealth encounter

   C) The patient's preference for telehealth over in-person visits

   D) The cost of the telehealth technology used

2. Documenting patient consent for telehealth services is:

   A) Optional, based on the provider's discretion

   B) Required only for video conferencing

   C) Crucial for all telehealth encounters

   D) Necessary only for international patients

3. Technical issues during a telehealth visit should be:

A) Ignored if they don't severely impact the session

B) Documented, including their impact on the consultation

C) Only reported to the IT department

D) Fixed by the patient before the visit

4. In telehealth documentation, noting the limitations of clinical assessments is important because:

A) It excuses the provider from any responsibility

B) It identifies areas for technological improvement

C) It acknowledges aspects of care that may require in-person follow-up

D) It shifts liability to the telehealth platform provider

5. Follow-up care instructions in telehealth documentation should be:

A) Less detailed than in-person visit instructions

B) The same as if the patient were seen in person

C) Only provided verbally

D) Sent via email instead of being documented

6. The privacy and security measures taken during a telehealth visit:

A) Need not be documented if standard protocols are followed

B) Should be documented, especially the use of encrypted communication

C) Are the responsibility of the patient

D) Only apply to certain types of telehealth technologies

7. The use of standardized templates in EHRs for telehealth documentation:

A) Is discouraged in favor of free text entries

B) Can improve consistency and completeness

C) Limits the provider's ability to document effectively

D) Is only useful for billing purposes

8. Consent for telehealth services typically covers:

A) Only the current visit

B) All future healthcare interactions

C) The use of technology and acknowledgment of its limitations

D) Consent for all medical treatments, irrespective of modality

9. When documenting a telehealth encounter, it's important to include:

  A) A description of the patient's home

  B) The patient's vital signs, even if self-reported

  C) The names of all family members present

  D) The provider's personal opinion on telehealth

10. A key advantage of telehealth documented in EHRs is:

  A) Reducing the need for patient consent

  B) Enhancing coordination of care across providers

  C) Completely replacing in-person visits

  D) Making healthcare more expensive but accessible

Answers:

1. B) The modality of the telehealth encounter

2. C) Crucial for all telehealth encounters

3. B) Documented, including their impact on the consultation

4. C) It acknowledges aspects of care that may require in-person follow-up

5. B) The same as if the patient were seen in person

6. B) Should be documented, especially the use of encrypted communication

7. B) Can improve consistency and completeness

8. C) The use of technology and acknowledgment of its limitations

9. B) The patient's vital signs, even if self-reported

10. B) Enhancing coordination of care across providers

Chapter 8: Training and Education for Documentation Specialists

8.1 Essential Skills and Competencies

Documentation specialists play a critical role in healthcare settings, ensuring the accuracy, completeness, and compliance of clinical documentation. Their work supports high-quality patient care, facilitates billing and reimbursement, and ensures adherence to regulatory requirements. To excel in this field, documentation specialists must possess a blend of technical skills, domain knowledge, and soft skills. This section outlines the essential skills and competencies required for success in this role.

Technical Proficiency

- **Understanding of Medical Terminology and Anatomy**: A foundational understanding of medical terminology, anatomy, and physiology is crucial for accurately interpreting and documenting clinical information.

- **Proficiency in Electronic Health Records (EHR) Systems**: Mastery of EHR systems, including navigation, data entry, and the use of templates and coding tools, is essential for efficient documentation.

- **Knowledge of Coding and Billing Practices**: Familiarity with ICD, CPT, and other coding systems, as well as an understanding of billing processes, supports accurate and compliant documentation for reimbursement purposes.

Regulatory Knowledge

- **Compliance with Healthcare Regulations**: Documentation specialists must be well-versed in healthcare regulations, including HIPAA, HITECH, and other laws affecting patient privacy and data security. They should understand the implications of these regulations for clinical documentation and patient care.

- **Accreditation Standards**: Awareness of accreditation standards from organizations such as The Joint Commission or NCQA is important for ensuring that documentation practices meet or exceed quality benchmarks.

Communication and Interpersonal Skills

- **Effective Communication**: Clear and effective communication with healthcare providers, coding staff, and other team members is vital for resolving documentation issues, providing feedback, and ensuring a cohesive approach to patient care.

- **Teamwork and Collaboration**: The ability to work collaboratively within interdisciplinary teams, including the capacity to negotiate and resolve conflicts, is essential for documentation specialists.

- **Critical Thinking and Problem-Solving**: Documentation specialists must be able to analyze complex information, identify documentation gaps or inconsistencies, and develop solutions to improve documentation quality and accuracy.

Continuous Learning and Adaptability

- **Commitment to Ongoing Education**: The healthcare landscape is continually evolving, with changes in medical practices, technologies, and regulations. Documentation specialists must be committed to ongoing learning and professional development.

- **Adaptability**: The ability to adapt to new technologies, workflows, and best practices is crucial for staying effective in the role of a documentation specialist.

Attention to Detail

- **Accuracy and Precision**: Given the impact of documentation on patient care and legal compliance, attention to detail is critical. Documentation specialists must ensure that all clinical information is accurately captured and reflects the care provided.

Conclusion

The role of a documentation specialist requires a diverse set of skills and competencies, spanning technical proficiency, regulatory knowledge, communication abilities, and a commitment to continuous improvement. By cultivating these essential skills, documentation specialists can significantly contribute to the efficiency, quality, and compliance of healthcare documentation, ultimately supporting the delivery of high-quality patient care.

8.2 Designing Effective Training Programs

For documentation specialists and healthcare providers alike, ongoing education and training are essential for maintaining high standards of clinical documentation. Designing effective training programs is crucial to ensuring that staff are well-versed in the latest documentation practices, technologies, and regulatory requirements. A well-structured training program can enhance accuracy, efficiency, and compliance, ultimately improving patient care and organizational performance. Here are key components and strategies for developing successful training programs in clinical documentation.

Needs Assessment

Begin with a comprehensive needs assessment to identify the specific knowledge and skill gaps among your staff. This assessment could involve analyzing documentation errors, conducting surveys or interviews with staff, and reviewing regulatory updates or new technology implementations that impact documentation practices. The findings will guide the development of targeted training objectives.

Customized Content

Develop training content that is tailored to the unique needs of your audience, whether they are new hires, experienced documentation specialists, or healthcare providers from various specialties. The content should cover a range of topics, including medical terminology, EHR system functionality, coding standards, regulatory compliance, and best practices in documentation. Incorporate real-world scenarios and examples to make the training relevant and engaging.

Interactive and Engaging Methods

To maximize the effectiveness of the training, employ a variety of teaching methods that cater to different learning styles. Interactive workshops, hands-on EHR system demonstrations, and group discussions can enhance engagement and retention. Consider incorporating gamification elements, such as quizzes or simulations, to make learning more interactive and enjoyable.

Expert Instructors

Engage knowledgeable instructors who are experts in clinical documentation and familiar with the latest trends and technologies. Instructors should be adept at communicating complex information clearly and able to answer questions and provide feedback. Guest speakers from regulatory bodies or industry leaders can also add valuable insights and perspectives.

Blended Learning Approach

A blended learning approach, combining in-person sessions with online modules, can offer flexibility and accommodate different learning paces. Online resources, such as video tutorials, webinars, and e-learning modules, allow participants to revisit materials as needed and engage in self-directed learning.

Ongoing Support and Resources

Provide ongoing support and resources beyond the initial training sessions. This could include access to online reference materials, forums for asking questions, and regular updates on documentation standards and regulatory changes. Establishing a mentorship program or a help desk can also offer additional support to staff as they apply their learning in practice.

Evaluation and Feedback

Incorporate mechanisms for evaluating the effectiveness of the training program, including pre- and post-training assessments, participant surveys, and performance metrics. Feedback from participants can inform continuous improvements to the training content and delivery methods.

Conclusion

Designing effective training programs for clinical documentation is a dynamic process that requires attention to the needs of the staff, the use of engaging teaching methods, and the provision of ongoing support. By investing in comprehensive and customized training, healthcare organizations can empower their staff to achieve excellence in documentation, enhancing the quality of care, compliance, and operational efficiency.

8.3 Certification and Continuing Education

In the rapidly evolving field of healthcare documentation, certification and continuing education are critical pathways for documentation specialists and healthcare providers to demonstrate their expertise, stay updated on the latest industry standards, and enhance their professional development. These educational pursuits not only contribute to personal career growth but also significantly impact the quality of patient care and organizational compliance with healthcare regulations.

Importance of Certification

- **Professional Recognition**: Certification offers documentation specialists and healthcare providers formal recognition of their expertise and commitment to excellence in clinical documentation. It validates their knowledge and skills, enhancing their credibility and professional standing.

- **Compliance and Quality Assurance**: Certified professionals are knowledgeable about the latest compliance standards and best practices in documentation. Their expertise helps ensure that healthcare organizations meet regulatory requirements and maintain high-quality documentation.

- **Career Advancement**: Certification can open doors to career advancement opportunities, including leadership roles in clinical documentation, health information management, and quality improvement initiatives. It often leads to greater job mobility and higher compensation.

Popular Certification Programs

Several organizations offer certification programs relevant to clinical documentation improvement (CDI) and health information management (HIM), including:

- **Certified Clinical Documentation Specialist (CCDS)**: Offered by the Association of Clinical Documentation Improvement Specialists (ACDIS), this certification is designed for CDI professionals seeking to validate their expertise.

- **Registered Health Information Administrator (RHIA)** and **Registered Health Information Technician (RHIT)**: Offered by the American Health Information Management Association (AHIMA), these certifications focus on health information management and the use of patient data in healthcare decision-making.

- **Certified Professional Coder (CPC)**: Offered by the American Academy of Professional Coders (AAPC), this certification is geared towards medical coders seeking to demonstrate their proficiency in coding patient medical records for billing purposes.

Continuing Education

- **Staying Current**: The healthcare industry is characterized by constant changes in regulations, technologies, and best practices. Continuing education enables documentation specialists to stay current with these changes, ensuring that their skills and knowledge remain relevant.

- **Skill Enhancement**: Through workshops, seminars, webinars, and online courses, professionals can deepen their expertise in specific areas, such as advanced coding techniques, EHR optimization, and legal aspects of healthcare documentation.

- **Networking Opportunities**: Continuing education events often provide opportunities to connect with peers, experts, and industry leaders. These networking opportunities can lead to professional collaborations, mentorship relationships, and insights into emerging trends in healthcare documentation.

Conclusion

Certification and continuing education are indispensable for documentation specialists and healthcare providers aiming to excel in their roles and contribute to the advancement of healthcare quality and compliance. By pursuing these educational pathways, professionals can ensure that they remain at the forefront of their field, equipped with the knowledge and skills necessary to meet the challenges of modern healthcare documentation.

8.4 Exercise: 10 MCQs with Answers at the End

Let's create a set of 10 multiple-choice questions (MCQs) focusing on the content covered in Chapter 8, which deals with training, education, certification, and continuing education for documentation specialists. This exercise is designed to reinforce key concepts and assess understanding.

1. What is the primary purpose of certification for documentation specialists?

   A) To reduce the workload of healthcare providers

   B) To formalize objections to new documentation practices

C) To recognize professional expertise and commitment to excellence

D) To eliminate the need for continuing education

2. Which certification is specifically designed for Clinical Documentation Improvement professionals?

A) RHIA

B) CPC

C) CCDS

D) RHIT

3. Continuing education for documentation specialists is important because it:

A) Allows them to avoid new regulatory requirements

B) Ensures their skills and knowledge remain relevant in a changing industry

C) Decreases their value within the healthcare team

D) Simplifies the documentation process to basic levels

4. A significant benefit of ongoing training for documentation specialists includes:

A) Decreasing collaboration with healthcare providers

B) Increasing documentation errors for learning purposes

C) Enhancing accuracy, efficiency, and compliance in documentation

D) Limiting their understanding to a single area of expertise

5. What type of learning approach combines in-person sessions with online modules?

A) Traditional learning

B) Blended learning

C) Isolated learning

D) Passive learning

6. The RHIT certification is offered by which organization?

A) ACDIS

B) AHIMA

C) AAPC

D) AMA

7. Effective training programs for clinical documentation should NOT:

A) Be tailored to the unique needs of the audience

B) Utilize a variety of interactive teaching methods

C) Exclude real-world scenarios and examples

D) Engage knowledgeable instructors

8. Which is not a direct benefit of professional certification in healthcare documentation?

A) Automatic promotion to leadership roles

B) Professional recognition

C) Enhanced credibility and professional standing

D) Career advancement opportunities

9. Why is adaptability considered an essential skill for documentation specialists?

A) It allows them to avoid learning new technologies

B) It enables them to maintain old documentation practices

C) It helps them adjust to new technologies, workflows, and best practices

D) It encourages them to work in isolation

10. Networking opportunities in continuing education can lead to:

A) Decreased professional collaborations

B) Diminished professional development

C) Insights into emerging trends in healthcare documentation

D) Reduced need for professional certification

Answers:

1. C) To recognize professional expertise and commitment to excellence

2. C) CCDS

3. B) Ensures their skills and knowledge remain relevant in a changing industry

4. C) Enhancing accuracy, efficiency, and compliance in documentation

5. B) Blended learning

6. B) AHIMA

7. C) Exclude real-world scenarios and examples

8. A) Automatic promotion to leadership roles

9. C) It helps them adjust to new technologies, workflows, and best practices

10. C) Insights into emerging trends in healthcare documentation

Chapter 9: Quality Assurance in Clinical Documentation

9.1 Implementing Quality Assurance Programs

Quality assurance (QA) in clinical documentation is crucial for maintaining high standards of patient care, ensuring regulatory compliance, and optimizing billing processes. Implementing an effective QA program involves systematic monitoring, evaluation, and improvement of documentation practices within a healthcare organization. This section outlines the key steps and considerations for establishing a robust QA program for clinical documentation.

Define Quality Standards and Objectives

The first step in implementing a QA program is to define clear quality standards and objectives based on industry best practices, regulatory requirements, and organizational goals. These standards should address the accuracy, completeness, timeliness, and compliance of clinical documentation. Setting measurable objectives allows for the assessment of the program's effectiveness over time.

Establish a QA Team

Forming a dedicated QA team is essential for the oversight and management of the QA program. This team should include clinical documentation specialists, healthcare providers, coding professionals, and representatives from the quality management department. The diversity of the team ensures a comprehensive approach to improving documentation practices across the organization.

Develop Review Processes

The QA team should develop standardized review processes for evaluating clinical documentation. This could involve random audits of patient records, targeted reviews based on identified risk areas, or periodic assessments of specific departments or services. The review process should include criteria for evaluating documentation against the defined quality standards.

Training and Education

Ongoing training and education are vital components of a QA program. Healthcare staff should be regularly updated on documentation standards, changes in regulatory requirements, and best practices in clinical documentation. Training programs can be tailored to address common documentation errors and areas for improvement identified through QA reviews.

Feedback and Reporting Mechanisms

Effective feedback and reporting mechanisms are crucial for communicating the findings of documentation reviews to healthcare providers and other relevant staff. Constructive feedback helps individuals understand documentation deficiencies and how to correct them. Regular reports on the QA program's outcomes, including trends in documentation quality and areas of success, foster a culture of continuous improvement.

Utilize Technology

Leveraging technology, such as electronic health records (EHRs) and clinical documentation improvement (CDI) software, can enhance the QA process. These tools can automate aspects of the review process, provide real-time alerts for documentation errors, and offer analytics for tracking improvements over time.

Continuous Improvement

Quality assurance in clinical documentation is an ongoing process. The QA team should regularly review the effectiveness of the program, incorporating feedback from healthcare providers, updates in regulations, and advancements in documentation practices. Continuous monitoring and adjustment of the QA program ensure it remains aligned with the organization's goals and the evolving landscape of healthcare.

Conclusion

Implementing a quality assurance program for clinical documentation is a strategic investment in the quality of patient care and the operational efficiency of healthcare organizations. By establishing clear standards, engaging a multidisciplinary team, and fostering a culture of continuous improvement, organizations can ensure their clinical documentation meets the highest standards of accuracy, completeness, and compliance.

9.2 Metrics for Measuring Documentation Quality

Evaluating the quality of clinical documentation is essential for healthcare organizations aiming to improve patient care, ensure regulatory compliance, and optimize reimbursement processes. By establishing clear metrics for measuring documentation quality, organizations can identify areas of strength and opportunities for improvement. This section discusses key metrics that are pivotal in assessing the effectiveness and quality of clinical documentation.

Accuracy

- **Correctness of Patient Information**: This metric evaluates the precision in documenting patient identification details, medical history, diagnoses, treatments administered, and outcomes. Accuracy is fundamental to patient safety and effective care coordination.

- **Consistency Across Records**: Measures the consistency of patient information across various documents and systems. Inconsistencies may lead to errors in patient care and billing.

Completeness

- **Inclusion of All Relevant Data**: Ensures that the documentation includes comprehensive details of the patient's condition, the care provided, and the outcomes. It evaluates whether the documentation meets the requirements for clinical, legal, and billing purposes.

- **Documentation of Every Patient Encounter**: Assesses whether every interaction with the patient, including consultations, procedures, and follow-up visits, is recorded in the patient's health record.

Timeliness

- **Promptness of Documentation**: Measures the speed with which clinical encounters are documented in the patient's record. Timely documentation ensures that information is available when needed for patient care and decision-making.

- **Up-to-date Patient Records**: Evaluates whether patient records are regularly updated to reflect the current state of the patient's condition and care plan.

Clarity and Readability

- **Legibility of Records**: For handwritten notes, this metric assesses how easily the text can be read. In the context of electronic records, it evaluates the organization and presentation of information.

- **Use of Standardized Language and Terminology**: Measures the use of standardized medical terminology and abbreviations, which is crucial for clear communication among healthcare professionals.

Compliance with Legal and Regulatory Standards

- **Adherence to Documentation Regulations**: Evaluates compliance with healthcare regulations, such as HIPAA in the United States, which governs the privacy and security of patient information.

- **Alignment with Coding and Billing Guidelines**: Assesses the documentation's compliance with coding standards and billing guidelines, crucial for accurate reimbursement.

Patient-Centeredness

- **Inclusion of Patient Preferences and Goals**: Measures how well the documentation reflects patient preferences, goals, and involvement in care decisions. This metric underscores the importance of patient-centered care.

Interdisciplinary Communication

- **Effectiveness in Facilitating Care Coordination**: Assesses the documentation's role in promoting seamless communication and coordination among different healthcare professionals involved in the patient's care.

Utilization and Efficiency

- **Reduction in Duplicate Tests and Procedures**: Evaluates how effective documentation is in reducing unnecessary repeat tests and procedures, contributing to healthcare efficiency and cost reduction.

Conclusion

By employing these metrics, healthcare organizations can systematically evaluate and monitor the quality of clinical documentation. This process not only highlights areas for improvement but also contributes to enhancing patient care, ensuring compliance, and optimizing operational processes. Continuous assessment and refinement of documentation practices, guided by these metrics, are essential for maintaining high standards of healthcare delivery.

9.3 Feedback and Improvement Cycles

Feedback and improvement cycles are fundamental components of quality assurance in clinical documentation. These cycles create a structured approach for continuous evaluation, feedback, and enhancement of documentation practices, ensuring they meet the highest standards of accuracy, completeness, and compliance. Implementing effective feedback and improvement cycles involves several key steps, fostering a culture of continuous learning and adaptation within healthcare organizations.

Identifying Areas for Improvement

The first step in the cycle involves systematically identifying areas where clinical documentation can be enhanced. This may be achieved through regular audits, peer reviews, and analysis of metrics for measuring documentation quality. Technology, such as electronic health record (EHR) systems with built-in analytics, can also provide valuable insights into documentation practices, highlighting inconsistencies, gaps, or trends that require attention.

Gathering and Analyzing Feedback

Feedback is a critical component of the improvement cycle. This feedback can come from a variety of sources, including healthcare providers, documentation specialists, coding and billing professionals, and even patients. Surveys, interviews, and suggestion boxes are effective tools for gathering feedback. Analyzing this feedback helps to understand the underlying causes of documentation issues and to prioritize areas for improvement.

Developing and Implementing Action Plans

Based on the identified areas for improvement and the feedback received, the next step is to develop action plans. These plans should outline specific strategies for addressing the issues identified, assign responsibilities, and set timelines for implementation. Action plans might include targeted training programs, updates to documentation templates or guidelines, enhancements to EHR systems, or changes to workflows to reduce documentation burdens on healthcare providers.

Providing Targeted Training and Support

Education and training are crucial for implementing changes in documentation practices. Targeted training sessions can address specific areas of concern, update staff on new documentation standards or technologies, and reinforce best practices. Providing ongoing support, such as access to documentation specialists or help desks, can assist staff in adapting to changes and overcoming challenges in real-time.

Monitoring Progress and Measuring Impact

After implementing the action plans, it's important to monitor progress and measure the impact of the changes on documentation quality. Revisiting the metrics for measuring documentation quality can provide objective data on improvements or highlight areas that need further attention. This step closes the feedback and improvement cycle and sets the stage for the next cycle of evaluation and enhancement.

Encouraging a Culture of Continuous Improvement

For feedback and improvement cycles to be effective, healthcare organizations must foster a culture that values continuous improvement, open communication, and collaborative problem-solving. Recognizing and rewarding improvements in documentation practices can motivate staff and reinforce the importance of high-quality clinical documentation.

Conclusion

Feedback and improvement cycles are essential for maintaining and enhancing the quality of clinical documentation. By systematically identifying areas for improvement, gathering and analyzing feedback, developing and implementing action plans, and monitoring progress, healthcare organizations can ensure their documentation practices support the highest standards of patient care, regulatory compliance, and operational efficiency. Encouraging a culture of continuous improvement empowers staff to contribute to the ongoing enhancement of documentation practices, benefiting patients, providers, and the organization as a whole.

9.4 Exercise: 10 MCQs with Answers at the End

Let's create a set of 10 multiple-choice questions (MCQs) based on the content of Chapter 9, focusing on implementing quality assurance programs, metrics for measuring documentation quality, and the process of feedback and improvement cycles in clinical documentation. This exercise aims to reinforce key concepts and assess understanding.

1. What is the primary goal of implementing quality assurance programs in clinical documentation?

   A) To reduce the workload of healthcare providers

   B) To enhance patient care and ensure regulatory compliance

   C) To limit the use of electronic health records

   D) To increase the complexity of documentation processes

2. A key metric for measuring the quality of clinical documentation is:

   A) The number of pages in a patient's file

   B) The speed at which documents are filed

   C) Accuracy and correctness of patient information

D) The color scheme of the documentation system

3. An effective quality assurance program in clinical documentation should NOT:

A) Ignore feedback from healthcare providers

B) Define clear quality standards and objectives

C) Employ a dedicated quality assurance team

D) Develop standardized review processes

4. Which of the following is NOT a common source of feedback for improving clinical documentation?

A) Patient surveys

B) External advertisements

C) Healthcare providers

D) Coding and billing professionals

5. Continuous improvement in clinical documentation is best achieved through:

A) Avoiding changes to established practices

B) Implementing feedback and improvement cycles

C) Decreasing communication among staff

D) Increasing documentation workload for providers

6. In the context of clinical documentation, clarity and readability are measured by:

A) The length of the documents

B) Use of standardized language and terminology

C) Number of acronyms used

D) Frequency of document updates

7. Timeliness in clinical documentation is important because it:

A) Allows for slower patient care

B) Ensures information is available when needed for decision-making

C) Makes documents harder to read over time

D) Reduces the need for electronic health records

8. A significant challenge in quality assurance for clinical documentation is:

A) Having too few documentation standards

B) The rapid pace of regulatory changes and technology advancements

C) Too much feedback from patients

D) The simplicity of the documentation process

9. The role of technology in the quality assurance of clinical documentation includes:

   A) Reducing the accuracy of records

   B) Providing analytics to track improvements

   C) Eliminating the need for human oversight

   D) Decreasing the security of patient information

10. Effective training and support for clinical documentation should:

   A) Focus solely on new staff members

   B) Avoid addressing specific documentation issues

   C) Be based on identified areas for improvement

   D) Discourage the use of electronic resources

Answers:

1. B) To enhance patient care and ensure regulatory compliance

2. C) Accuracy and correctness of patient information

3. A) Ignore feedback from healthcare providers

4. B) External advertisements

5. B) Implementing feedback and improvement cycles

6. B) Use of standardized language and terminology

7. B) Ensures information is available when needed for decision-making

8. B) The rapid pace of regulatory changes and technology advancements

9. B) Providing analytics to track improvements

10. C) Be based on identified areas for improvement

Chapter 10: Communication and Collaboration

10.1 Effective Communication Strategies

Effective communication is the cornerstone of high-quality healthcare delivery, enabling seamless coordination among healthcare providers and ensuring that patients receive comprehensive and coherent care. In the context of clinical documentation, clear and effective communication strategies are vital for capturing accurate and complete patient information, reducing errors, and facilitating collaborative decision-making. This section explores key strategies for enhancing communication within healthcare settings.

Active Listening

Active listening involves fully concentrating on what is being said rather than passively hearing the speaker's words. It includes paying attention to the speaker's body language, providing feedback, and refraining from interrupting. In clinical settings, active listening can improve the accuracy of patient information collected and ensure that all team members' perspectives are considered in care decisions.

Standardized Communication Tools

Implementing standardized communication tools and protocols, such as SBAR (Situation, Background, Assessment, Recommendation), can help ensure that critical patient information is conveyed clearly and concisely between providers. These tools provide a framework for reporting patient information, facilitating consistent and efficient exchanges.

Closed-Loop Communication

Closed-loop communication is a technique used to ensure that information is understood correctly by having the receiver repeat back what they have heard to the sender. This method is particularly useful in high-stakes environments like healthcare, where misunderstandings can lead to errors in patient care.

Multidisciplinary Team Meetings

Regular multidisciplinary team meetings provide an opportunity for healthcare providers from various specialties to come together, discuss patient care, and share information. These meetings foster a collaborative approach to patient care, ensuring that all aspects of a patient's health are considered and documented.

Leveraging Technology

Technology, such as electronic health records (EHRs) and secure messaging platforms, can significantly enhance communication among healthcare providers. EHRs allow for real-time access to patient information, while secure messaging platforms enable quick and efficient exchanges between team members. Adopting these technologies can improve the accuracy and timeliness of clinical documentation.

Patient-Centered Communication

Engaging patients in discussions about their care and encouraging them to ask questions and express concerns can lead to more accurate and comprehensive documentation. Patient-centered communication not only improves the quality of care but also enhances patient satisfaction and adherence to treatment plans.

Cultural Competence

Being culturally competent and sensitive to the diverse backgrounds and needs of patients is essential for effective communication. Healthcare providers should be trained to recognize and respect cultural differences, which can influence how patients perceive their care, communicate their needs, and understand health information.

Feedback and Continuous Improvement

Creating a culture that values feedback and continuous improvement can enhance communication practices. Encouraging feedback from patients, family members, and healthcare providers about communication effectiveness can identify areas for enhancement.

Conclusion

Effective communication strategies are essential for ensuring high-quality clinical documentation and patient care. By fostering active listening, utilizing standardized communication tools, leveraging technology, and promoting a collaborative and patient-centered approach, healthcare organizations can improve the accuracy, efficiency, and effectiveness of their communication practices. Continuous evaluation and improvement of communication strategies are key to adapting to the evolving needs of healthcare delivery.

10.2 Interdisciplinary Collaboration for Patient Care

Interdisciplinary collaboration in healthcare involves the cooperative integration of expertise from various healthcare professionals to provide comprehensive patient care. This collaborative approach is crucial for addressing the complex and multifaceted needs of patients, particularly those with chronic conditions or requiring complex interventions. Effective interdisciplinary collaboration enhances patient outcomes, improves the efficiency of care delivery, and contributes to more satisfying work environments for healthcare professionals. Here's how it can be effectively implemented and its impact on patient care.

Benefits of Interdisciplinary Collaboration

- **Comprehensive Care**: Brings together diverse expertise to address all aspects of a patient's health, ensuring a holistic approach to treatment and care planning.

- **Improved Patient Outcomes**: Studies have shown that interdisciplinary collaboration can lead to better health outcomes, including reduced hospital readmissions, improved management of chronic diseases, and higher patient satisfaction.

- **Enhanced Communication**: Fosters clear and open communication channels among team members, reducing the potential for errors and enhancing the continuity of care.

- **Increased Efficiency**: Coordination among various healthcare providers can streamline care processes, reduce duplicative assessments, and expedite interventions, saving time and resources.

Strategies for Enhancing Interdisciplinary Collaboration

- **Define Clear Roles and Responsibilities**: Clearly outlining the role of each team member helps to avoid overlaps in duties and ensures that all aspects of patient care are covered. Understanding each member's expertise and responsibilities fosters mutual respect and trust.

- **Regular Team Meetings**: Scheduled meetings provide opportunities for team members to discuss patient cases, share insights, and develop cohesive care plans. These meetings can be in-person or virtual, leveraging technology to facilitate communication.

- **Shared Goals and Objectives**: Establishing common goals for patient care encourages team members to work together towards achieving these objectives, focusing on patient-centered outcomes.

- **Cross-disciplinary Training**: Providing team members with training on the basics of each other's roles and perspectives can enhance understanding and appreciation of diverse professional contributions to patient care.

- **Use of Collaborative Tools**: Electronic health records (EHRs), shared documentation platforms, and other collaborative tools can facilitate the seamless exchange of patient information and care plans among interdisciplinary team members.

- **Conflict Resolution Mechanisms**: Implementing strategies for resolving disagreements or conflicts constructively is essential for maintaining a collaborative team environment. This might include regular debriefings or mediation by an impartial third party.

- **Patient and Family Involvement**: Engaging patients and their families as active members of the healthcare team can provide valuable insights into care preferences, contributing to more tailored and effective care strategies.

Conclusion

Interdisciplinary collaboration in patient care is a cornerstone of modern healthcare delivery, ensuring that patient care is comprehensive, efficient, and tailored to individual needs. By implementing strategies that foster collaboration among diverse healthcare professionals, healthcare organizations can enhance patient outcomes, improve the quality of care, and create more fulfilling work environments for staff. As healthcare becomes increasingly complex, the importance of effective interdisciplinary collaboration will continue to grow, underscoring the need for ongoing efforts to strengthen these collaborative practices.

10.3 Navigating Conflicts and Miscommunications

In the multidisciplinary nature of healthcare, conflicts and miscommunications are inevitable. Differences in perspectives, misunderstandings, and the high-stress environment can lead to disputes among healthcare professionals, potentially impacting patient care. Navigating these challenges effectively is crucial for maintaining a collaborative, respectful, and productive working environment. This section explores strategies for managing conflicts and miscommunications in healthcare settings.

Recognizing the Sources of Conflict

Understanding the root causes of conflicts is the first step towards resolution. Conflicts may arise from:

- **Role Ambiguities**: Unclear definitions of responsibilities can lead to overlaps or gaps in patient care.

- **Communication Breakdowns**: Misunderstandings or lack of information can result in disagreements on patient management strategies.

- **Differences in Professional Culture**: Diverse training backgrounds and professional cultures can lead to differing approaches to patient care.

- **Resource Limitations**: Constraints on time, personnel, or materials can heighten tensions among staff.

Effective Strategies for Conflict Resolution

- **Open Communication**: Encourage open dialogue where team members can express concerns and perspectives in a respectful and constructive manner. Active listening and empathy can help de-escalate tensions.

- **Clarification of Roles and Expectations**: Clearly defining roles, responsibilities, and expectations can prevent many conflicts related to role ambiguity.

- **Conflict Resolution Training**: Providing training on conflict resolution techniques can equip healthcare professionals with the skills to manage disputes effectively.

- **Seeking Mediation**: In cases where conflicts cannot be resolved internally, seeking assistance from a neutral third party or a mediator can help find common ground and resolve the dispute.

Mitigating Miscommunications

Miscommunications can lead to errors in patient care and inefficiencies in healthcare delivery. Strategies to mitigate miscommunications include:

- **Standardized Communication Protocols**: Implementing standardized tools and protocols, like SBAR (Situation, Background, Assessment, Recommendation), can enhance the clarity and consistency of communication.

- **Documentation Best Practices**: Ensuring accurate and timely documentation in patient records can reduce misunderstandings and provide a reliable source of patient information.

- **Regular Team Meetings**: Holding regular interdisciplinary team meetings allows for real-time updates and clarifications on patient care plans, reducing the risk of miscommunications.

- **Training on Communication Skills**: Providing training on effective communication techniques can improve the ability of healthcare professionals to convey and receive information clearly.

Promoting a Culture of Collaboration and Respect

- **Fostering Mutual Respect**: Cultivating an environment of mutual respect among healthcare professionals, regardless of their roles or specialties, can create a foundation for effective collaboration and conflict resolution.

- **Team-building Activities**: Engaging in team-building activities can strengthen relationships among team members, improving communication and reducing the likelihood of conflicts.

- **Recognition and Valuation of Contributions**: Acknowledging and valuing the contributions of all team members can promote a sense of belonging and respect, which is critical for resolving conflicts constructively.

Conclusion

Effectively navigating conflicts and miscommunications is essential for maintaining a harmonious and productive healthcare environment. By implementing clear communication strategies, conflict resolution training, and fostering a culture of collaboration and respect, healthcare organizations can mitigate the impact of disputes and misunderstandings, ultimately enhancing patient care and team cohesion.

10.4 Exercise: 10 MCQs with Answers at the End

Let's create a set of 10 multiple-choice questions (MCQs) based on the content of Chapter 10, focusing on effective communication strategies, interdisciplinary collaboration for patient care, and navigating conflicts and miscommunications. This exercise aims to reinforce key concepts and assess understanding.

1. Active listening in healthcare communication is important because it:

  A) Ensures that messages are broadcasted loudly.

  B) Allows the listener to plan what to say next.

  C) Helps in fully understanding the speaker's message.

  D) Decreases the time needed for consultations.

2. Which of the following is a standardized communication tool in healthcare?

 A) SBAR (Situation, Background, Assessment, Recommendation)

  B) ASAP (As Soon As Possible)

  C) FYI (For Your Information)

  D) LOL (Laugh Out Loud)

3. Closed-loop communication enhances healthcare by:

A) Creating more paperwork for providers.

B) Ensuring information is correctly understood.

C) Limiting dialogue between team members.

D) Making communication more complex.

4. The primary benefit of interdisciplinary team meetings is:

A) Reducing the frequency of patient visits.

B) Enhancing competition among healthcare providers.

C) Improving coordination of comprehensive patient care.

D) Simplifying medical terminology.

5. Leveraging technology, such as EHRs, in communication primarily helps to:

A) Increase manual record-keeping.

B) Isolate healthcare team members.

C) Improve the accuracy and timeliness of clinical documentation.

D) Complicate the billing process.

6. Patient-centered communication is crucial for:

A) Discouraging patients from asking questions.

B) Ensuring that only the healthcare provider's goals are met.

C) Enhancing patient satisfaction and adherence to treatment plans.

D) Reducing the need for follow-up appointments.

7. A common source of conflict in healthcare settings is:

A) Too much clarity in role definitions.

B) Excessive communication among team members.

C) Ambiguities in roles and responsibilities.

D) The absence of any resource limitations.

8. Effective strategies for conflict resolution include all EXCEPT:

A) Ignoring the conflict and hoping it resolves itself.

B) Encouraging open dialogue and active listening.

C) Seeking mediation from a neutral third party.

D) Clarifying roles and expectations.

9. Mitigating miscommunications can be achieved through:

A) Decreasing the use of standardized communication protocols.

B) Ensuring accurate and timely documentation in patient records.

C) Limiting the frequency of interdisciplinary team meetings.

D) Avoiding training on effective communication techniques.

10. Promoting a culture of collaboration and respect in healthcare involves:

  A) Only recognizing the contributions of senior team members.

  B) Fostering mutual respect among all team members.

  C) Discouraging team-building activities.

  D) Valuing competition over cooperation.

Answers:

1. C) Helps in fully understanding the speaker's message.

2. A) SBAR (Situation, Background, Assessment, Recommendation)

3. B) Ensuring information is correctly understood.

4. C) Improving coordination of comprehensive patient care.

5. C) Improve the accuracy and timeliness of clinical documentation.

6. C) Enhancing patient satisfaction and adherence to treatment plans.

7. C) Ambiguities in roles and responsibilities.

8. A) Ignoring the conflict and hoping it resolves itself.

9. B) Ensuring accurate and timely documentation in patient records.

10. B) Fostering mutual respect among all team members.

Chapter 11: Patient Engagement and Documentation

11.1 Empowering Patients Through Access to Their Records

Empowering patients by providing access to their health records is a transformative approach in healthcare that fosters greater patient engagement, improves health outcomes, and enhances the patient-provider relationship. This strategy recognizes patients as active participants in their care, rather than passive recipients. The accessibility of health records allows patients to better understand their health conditions, treatment plans, and care processes, ultimately contributing to more informed decision-making and self-management.

Benefits of Patient Access to Records

- **Increased Transparency**: Providing patients with access to their health records promotes transparency in healthcare delivery, helping patients to understand their health status and the care they receive.

- **Improved Communication**: Access to records can facilitate more effective communication between patients and healthcare providers, as patients can prepare questions and discuss their care plans more knowledgeably.

- **Enhanced Patient Safety**: Patients who review their records can help identify and correct errors or omissions, contributing to their safety.

- **Greater Patient Engagement**: Access to health information empowers patients to take an active role in managing their health, leading to better adherence to treatment plans and preventive measures.

- **Higher Satisfaction**: Patients who have access to their health information typically report higher satisfaction with their care, as it fosters a sense of partnership with their healthcare providers.

Implementing Patient Access

- **Electronic Health Records (EHRs) and Patient Portals**: Many EHR systems include patient portals that offer secure online access to health records. These portals can provide patients with real-time information, including lab results, medication lists, and visit summaries.

- **Educational Resources**: Accompanying health records with educational materials or links to reputable sources can help patients better understand their health conditions and treatments.

- **Privacy and Security**: Ensuring the privacy and security of patient information is paramount. Access must be provided in a manner that protects patient data from unauthorized access or breaches.

- **Support and Guidance**: Offering support for patients on how to access and use their health records is crucial. This might include training sessions, help desks, or instructional materials.

Challenges and Considerations

While there are many benefits to providing patients with access to their health records, there are also challenges to consider, including:

- **Digital Divide**: Not all patients may have the digital literacy or access required to use online health portals effectively.

- **Information Overload**: Some patients may feel overwhelmed by the medical information or terminology in their records.

- **Privacy Concerns**: Balancing transparency with the need to protect sensitive health information can be complex, especially in the context of mental health or adolescent care.

Conclusion

Empowering patients through access to their health records is a critical component of modern healthcare that promotes engagement, improves outcomes, and enhances the care experience. By implementing strategies that facilitate access while addressing potential challenges, healthcare providers can foster a more informed, engaged, and satisfied patient population.

11.2 Involving Patients in the Documentation Process

Involving patients in the clinical documentation process represents a shift towards more patient-centered care, recognizing patients as active partners in their healthcare journey. This involvement can vary from patients reviewing their records for accuracy to directly contributing information about their health status and treatment experiences. Such engagement not only enhances the accuracy and completeness of clinical documentation but also empowers patients, improving their satisfaction and outcomes.

Strategies for Involving Patients

- **Patient-Generated Health Data (PGHD)**: Encourage patients to contribute data they collect through health apps, wearables, or personal health diaries. This data can provide valuable insights into their daily health, activities, and response to treatments.

- **Patient Annotations**: Some electronic health record (EHR) systems allow patients to add annotations or comments to their records. These annotations can clarify information, note perceived errors, or provide additional context.

- **Pre-Visit Questionnaires**: Utilize pre-visit questionnaires to gather comprehensive health information from patients. This can help streamline the documentation process and ensure that important patient-reported information is captured.

- **Shared Decision-Making Tools**: Implement tools and processes that facilitate shared decision-making, allowing patients to actively participate in care planning. Documentation of these decisions can reflect a more accurate and collaborative care process.

Benefits of Patient Involvement

- **Enhanced Documentation Accuracy**: Direct input from patients can correct inaccuracies and fill gaps in the health record, leading to more reliable documentation.

- **Improved Patient Engagement**: Patients who are actively involved in the documentation process are more likely to be engaged in their care, leading to better adherence to treatment plans and improved health outcomes.

- **Empowered Patients**: Providing patients with a voice in their healthcare documentation empowers them and acknowledges their role in managing their health.

- **Strengthened Patient-Provider Relationship**: Collaborative documentation practices can strengthen the relationship between patients and providers, building trust and improving communication.

Challenges and Considerations

- **Privacy and Confidentiality**: Balancing patient involvement with the need to protect sensitive health information requires careful consideration and clear policies.

- **Information Overload**: Ensuring that patient contributions are valuable and relevant, without overwhelming the health record with unnecessary information, is crucial.

- **Health Literacy**: Patients with varying levels of health literacy may need additional support to contribute meaningfully to their records.

- **Technology Barriers**: Access to and familiarity with digital health tools can vary among patients, potentially limiting the feasibility of certain types of patient involvement.

Implementing Patient Involvement

Successful implementation of patient involvement in documentation requires:

- **Clear Guidelines and Training**: Provide clear guidelines for both patients and healthcare providers on how patients can contribute to their records. Training can help ensure that contributions are meaningful and constructive.

- **Support Systems**: Offer support systems, such as help desks or patient navigators, to assist patients in understanding how to access and interact with their health records.

- **Feedback Mechanisms**: Establish mechanisms for patients to provide feedback on the documentation process, facilitating continuous improvement.

Conclusion

Involving patients in the clinical documentation process is a forward-thinking approach that aligns with the principles of patient-centered care. By adopting strategies that enable and support patient contributions, healthcare providers can enhance the accuracy, completeness, and personal relevance of clinical documentation, leading to better patient engagement and healthcare outcomes.

11.3 Addressing Patient Concerns About Privacy

In an era where patient involvement in healthcare documentation is increasing, addressing concerns about privacy becomes paramount. As patients gain more access to their health records and contribute to their documentation, ensuring the confidentiality and security of their information is critical. This reassurance is not only a legal requirement but also essential for maintaining trust between patients and healthcare providers. This section explores strategies for addressing patient concerns about privacy in the context of clinical documentation.

Educating Patients on Privacy Protections

- **Inform Patients About Their Rights**: Patients should be informed about their rights regarding privacy and how their information is protected under laws such as the Health Insurance Portability and Accountability Act (HIPAA) in the United States or the General Data Protection Regulation (GDPR) in the European Union.

- **Explain Security Measures**: Clearly explain the security measures in place to protect patient information, including encryption, secure access protocols, and data breach response plans. Understanding these measures can reassure patients about the safety of their data.

Implementing Strict Access Controls

- **Role-based Access**: Ensure that access to patient records is limited to healthcare professionals directly involved in the patient's care. Role-based access controls can restrict access based on the staff member's role and necessity to know.

- **Audit Trails**: Maintain audit trails that log who accessed patient information, what was accessed, and when. Audit trails are crucial for monitoring access and detecting any unauthorized or inappropriate access to patient data.

Transparent Communication and Consent Processes

- **Informed Consent**: When involving patients in their documentation or collecting patient-generated health data (PGHD), obtain informed consent that explains how the information will be used, who will have access, and the patient's rights to access and amend their records.

- **Addressing Concerns**: Provide avenues for patients to express their privacy concerns, ask questions, and receive prompt, reassuring responses. This could include patient information hotlines, FAQ sections on patient portals, or direct discussions with healthcare providers.

Regular Review and Update of Privacy Policies

- **Stay Updated**: Regularly review and update privacy policies and practices to align with current laws, regulations, and technological advancements. Keeping policies up to date is essential for protecting patient information effectively.

- **Patient Notification**: Notify patients about any changes to privacy policies or practices, especially those that may affect how their information is used or shared. Transparency in policy changes reinforces trust and respect for patient privacy.

Technological Solutions

- **Secure Patient Portals**: Utilize secure patient portals for sharing information with patients. These portals should employ strong authentication methods to ensure that only the patient or authorized individuals can access the information.

- **Encryption**: Encrypt patient data both at rest and in transit to protect against unauthorized access or interception.

Conclusion

Addressing patient concerns about privacy is a critical aspect of modern healthcare, particularly as patients become more engaged with their health records and documentation. By educating patients, implementing strict access controls, maintaining transparent communication and consent processes, and utilizing technological solutions to secure data, healthcare providers can reassure patients about the confidentiality and safety of their information. These efforts are essential for maintaining patient trust and fostering a collaborative, patient-centered approach to healthcare.

11.4 Exercise: 10 MCQs with Answers at the End

Let's create a set of 10 multiple-choice questions (MCQs) based on the content of Chapter 11, focusing on empowering patients through access to their records, involving patients in the documentation process, addressing privacy concerns, and the overall theme of patient engagement and documentation. This exercise aims to reinforce key concepts and assess understanding.

1. Empowering patients through access to their health records can lead to:

A) Decreased patient satisfaction.

B) Increased transparency and patient engagement.

C) Reduced quality of care.

D) Higher rates of misinformation.

2. A primary benefit of involving patients in the documentation process is:

A) Increased workload for healthcare providers.

B) Enhanced documentation accuracy and completeness.

C) Decreased patient interest in their care.

D) More complex documentation processes.

3. Addressing patient concerns about privacy is crucial for:

A) Discouraging patients from accessing their records.

B) Maintaining trust between patients and healthcare providers.

C) Limiting the information shared with patients.

D) Increasing the complexity of healthcare services.

4. Which of the following is NOT a strategy for involving patients in their documentation?

A) Allowing patients to annotate their health records.

B) Encouraging patients to ignore their health data.

C) Utilizing pre-visit questionnaires.

D) Implementing shared decision-making tools.

5. Patient portals are used to:

A) Discourage patients from learning about their health conditions.

B) Provide secure online access to health records and information.

C) Reduce communication between patients and healthcare providers.

D) Increase the burden of documentation on patients.

6. Educating patients about their privacy rights involves informing them about:

A) The irrelevance of privacy laws.

B) Their rights under laws like HIPAA and GDPR.

C) How to avoid sharing their health information.

D) Ways to limit their access to healthcare.

7. Audit trails in patient health records are important for:

A) Tracking unauthorized access to patient information.

B) Decreasing transparency in healthcare.

C) Complicating the documentation process.

D) Reducing patient trust in healthcare providers.

8. Informed consent in the context of patient documentation is important for:

A) Ensuring patients are unaware of how their information is used.

B) Explaining how patient information will be used and shared.

C) Limiting patient access to their own health records.

D) Increasing unauthorized access to patient information.

9. A secure patient portal contributes to patient engagement by:

A) Limiting patient access to health information.

B) Providing real-time updates and facilitating communication.

C) Discouraging patients from participating in their care.

D) Exposing patient information to unauthorized users.

10. One challenge in providing patients with access to their health records is:

A) The unnecessary improvement in patient-provider communication.

B) The potential for information overload and misunderstanding.

C) Enhanced privacy and security of patient information.

D) Decreased patient interest in their healthcare.

Answers:

1. B) Increased transparency and patient engagement.

2. B) Enhanced documentation accuracy and completeness.

3. B) Maintaining trust between patients and healthcare providers.

4. B) Encouraging patients to ignore their health data.

5. B) Provide secure online access to health records and information.

6. B) Their rights under laws like HIPAA and GDPR.

7. A) Tracking unauthorized access to patient information.

8. B) Explaining how patient information will be used and shared.

9. B) Providing real-time updates and facilitating communication.

10. B) The potential for information overload and misunderstanding.

Chapter 12: Legal and Ethical Challenges

12.1 Navigating Complex Legal Scenarios

Healthcare professionals frequently encounter complex legal scenarios that impact clinical documentation and patient care. These scenarios can arise from regulatory requirements, patient privacy concerns, and the need for informed consent, among others. Navigating these legal intricacies is crucial for maintaining the trust of patients, ensuring compliance, and safeguarding the legal interests of healthcare providers and institutions. This section explores strategies for managing complex legal situations related to clinical documentation.

Understanding Regulatory Requirements

A thorough understanding of healthcare regulations is foundational. Professionals should be familiar with:

- **Health Insurance Portability and Accountability Act (HIPAA)**: Governs patient privacy and the security of health information in the U.S.

- **General Data Protection Regulation (GDPR)**: Regulates data protection and privacy in the European Union.

- **Local and State Laws**: May impose additional requirements on healthcare documentation and patient privacy.

Ensuring Informed Consent

Informed consent is a legal and ethical cornerstone of patient care, requiring clear communication about the risks, benefits, and alternatives of proposed treatments. Documentation of informed consent is critical and must detail the information provided to the patient, the patient's understanding, and their voluntary agreement to proceed.

Protecting Patient Privacy

Safeguarding patient privacy involves:

- **Implementing Secure Documentation Practices**: Utilizing secure, encrypted systems for storing and accessing patient records.

- **Limiting Access**: Ensuring that only authorized personnel have access to patient information, based on the principle of the minimum necessary use.

Dealing with Legal Requests for Information

Healthcare organizations may receive requests for patient information from legal entities. Handling these requests requires:

- **Verifying the Authority of the Request**: Confirming that the request comes from a legitimate legal source and specifies the information needed.

- **Ensuring Proper Authorization**: Releasing information only when appropriate legal documentation, such as subpoenas or court orders, is provided, or patient consent is obtained.

Maintaining Accurate and Timely Documentation

Accurate and timely documentation can protect healthcare providers in legal disputes by providing a clear, contemporaneous record of care provided. It's essential to:

- **Document Thoroughly**: Including all relevant patient interactions, decisions made, and the rationale for treatment choices.

- **Update Records Promptly**: Ensuring that patient records are current and reflect the latest care provided.

Ethical Considerations

Beyond legal compliance, ethical considerations should guide documentation practices, including:

- **Honesty and Integrity**: Ensuring that documentation is truthful and accurate.

- **Respecting Patient Autonomy**: Honoring patients' rights to access their information and make informed decisions about their care.

Training and Education

Ongoing training and education on legal issues in healthcare documentation are essential for keeping staff updated on laws, regulations, and best practices. This education can help prevent legal issues and enhance the quality of patient care.

Conclusion

Navigating complex legal scenarios in healthcare documentation requires a comprehensive understanding of laws and regulations, ethical principles, and practical strategies for compliance. By adhering to these guidelines, healthcare professionals can manage legal risks effectively while upholding high standards of patient care and confidentiality.

12.2 Ethical Decision-Making in Documentation

Ethical decision-making in clinical documentation involves navigating situations where the right course of action may not be clear-cut, requiring a balance between various ethical principles, professional standards, and patient interests. These situations can range from how to document sensitive patient information to addressing documentation errors. Here's how healthcare professionals can approach ethical decision-making in documentation to ensure that patient care and confidentiality are maintained without compromising professional integrity.

Core Ethical Principles in Documentation

- **Autonomy**: Respecting patient autonomy involves honoring their right to access and control their own health information. Documentation should accurately reflect the patient's health status and decisions regarding their care.

- **Beneficence**: This principle entails acting in the best interest of the patient. In documentation, this means ensuring that the information is complete and accurate to support optimal patient care.

- **Non-maleficence**: Avoiding harm is a critical consideration. Ethical documentation practices ensure that the information does not inadvertently harm the patient, whether through breaches of confidentiality or inaccuracies.

- **Justice**: This principle requires fair treatment of all patients. Documentation practices should not discriminate based on patient characteristics such as age, gender, race, or socioeconomic status.

Strategies for Ethical Decision-Making

- **Reflect on Ethical Principles**: When faced with a dilemma, consider how core ethical principles apply to the situation and use them as a guide for action.

- **Consult Guidelines and Policies**: Review professional guidelines, institutional policies, and legal requirements that may influence how certain information should be documented.

- **Seek Input from Colleagues**: Collaborative discussions with colleagues or an ethics committee can provide diverse perspectives and guidance on ethical issues.

- **Consider the Patient's Perspective**: When possible, involving the patient in decisions about how their information is documented can help address ethical concerns, especially those related to autonomy and privacy.

- **Document Transparently and Accurately**: Ensure that documentation reflects the truth about patient care, including any uncertainties or changes in the patient's condition. Transparent documentation supports ethical decision-making and patient care.

Common Ethical Challenges in Documentation

- **Handling Sensitive Information**: Deciding how to document sensitive aspects of a patient's health, such as mental health issues or substance use, requires careful consideration of privacy and potential stigma.

- **Addressing Documentation Errors**: Ethically managing errors in documentation involves correcting them transparently while ensuring that the original information and the correction are both clear and accessible.

- **Balancing Completeness with Relevance**: While comprehensive documentation is important, it's also necessary to ensure that the information included is relevant and does not violate the patient's privacy without reason.

Conclusion

Ethical decision-making in clinical documentation is complex, requiring careful consideration of ethical principles, professional standards, and patient interests. By adhering to ethical guidelines, consulting with colleagues, and focusing on transparent and accurate documentation, healthcare professionals can navigate these challenges effectively. Ultimately, ethical documentation practices support high-quality patient care, safeguard patient privacy, and maintain the integrity of the healthcare profession.

12.3 Confidentiality and Its Exceptions

Confidentiality is a cornerstone of the patient-healthcare provider relationship, underpinning trust and encouraging open communication. However, there are circumstances under which the ethical and legal obligation to maintain patient confidentiality may be overridden. Understanding these exceptions is crucial for healthcare professionals to navigate the delicate balance between respecting patient privacy and fulfilling other ethical or legal duties.

Understanding Confidentiality

Confidentiality involves keeping personal health information private unless the patient provides consent to disclose it. This principle is protected under laws like the Health Insurance Portability and Accountability Act (HIPAA) in the United States and similar regulations globally.

Standard Exceptions to Confidentiality

- **Risk of Harm to Self or Others**: If a patient poses a clear and immediate risk of serious harm to themselves or others, healthcare providers may have a duty to breach confidentiality to prevent that harm. This includes situations where patients express intentions of suicide, violence, or significant neglect.

- **Public Health Risks**: In the case of communicable diseases that pose significant public health risks, healthcare providers may be required to report cases to public health authorities to prevent the spread of disease.

- **Legal Requirements**: Legal proceedings may require healthcare providers to disclose patient information. This could be in response to court orders, subpoenas, or specific legal obligations to report certain conditions or incidents, such as gunshot wounds or signs of abuse.

- **Minors and Incapacity**: When patients are minors or lack the capacity to make informed decisions, healthcare providers may share relevant health information with parents, guardians, or legal representatives, always aiming to act in the patient's best interests.

Navigating Exceptions to Confidentiality

- **Minimize Breaches**: When breaching confidentiality, healthcare providers should disclose only the information necessary for the specific situation, maintaining privacy as much as possible.

- **Document Decisions**: Healthcare professionals should document their decisions to breach confidentiality, including the rationale and the information disclosed, ensuring a transparent record of their ethical and legal considerations.

- **Ethical Consultation**: In complex situations, seeking advice from ethics committees or legal counsel can provide valuable guidance on handling confidentiality exceptions.

- **Patient Communication**: Whenever possible, informing patients about the need to disclose their information can help maintain trust, even when confidentiality must be breached.

Educating Healthcare Professionals

Ongoing education and training on the principles of confidentiality and its exceptions are essential for healthcare professionals. This education helps ensure that staff are equipped to handle sensitive situations ethically and legally.

Conclusion

While confidentiality is a fundamental ethical and legal obligation in healthcare, exceptions exist for preventing harm, protecting public health, and complying with legal mandates. Healthcare professionals must navigate these exceptions thoughtfully, balancing the duty to protect patient privacy with broader ethical and societal obligations. Proper education, documentation, and ethical consultation are key to managing these complex scenarios effectively.

12.4 Exercise: 10 MCQs with Answers at the End

Let's create a set of 10 multiple-choice questions (MCQs) based on the content of Chapter 12, focusing on navigating complex legal scenarios, ethical decision-making in documentation, confidentiality and its exceptions, and the overall theme of legal and ethical challenges in clinical documentation. This exercise aims to reinforce key concepts and assess understanding.

1. The principle of confidentiality in healthcare is legally protected under:

A) GDPR in the European Union.

B) HIPAA in the United States.

C) Both A and B.

D) Neither A nor B.

2. An ethical obligation to breach confidentiality might arise when:

A) A patient requests complete privacy.

B) A patient poses a clear and immediate risk of serious harm to others.

C) There is a minor disagreement among healthcare providers.

D) A patient refuses treatment.

3. Effective strategies for ethical decision-making in documentation do NOT include:

A) Ignoring ethical principles to expedite care.

B) Reflecting on ethical principles applicable to the situation.

C) Consulting guidelines and policies.

D) Seeking input from colleagues.

4. Confidentiality can be legally overridden in the case of:

A) Routine treatment.

B) Communicable diseases with public health risks.

C) General dissatisfaction with care.

D) All personal health information requests from family.

5. Ethical decision-making in clinical documentation involves balancing:

A) The needs of the healthcare provider over the patient.

B) Financial considerations over patient safety.

C) Various ethical principles, professional standards, and patient interests.

D) The easiest course of action over the correct one.

6. Informed consent in documentation is crucial for:

A) Limiting the patient's knowledge about their condition.

B) Explaining how patient information will be used and shared.

C) Discouraging questions from the patient.

D) Reducing legal liability without improving understanding.

7. A healthcare professional may ethically disclose patient information without consent when:

A) The information is interesting or unusual.

B) It's convenient for administrative purposes.

C) Preventing significant harm to the patient or others.

D) The patient is uncooperative.

8. Confidentiality exceptions for minors typically allow disclosure to:

A) Any interested party.

B) Parents or legal guardians.

C) All healthcare workers, regardless of involvement in the case.

D) Media outlets for educational purposes.

9. When navigating complex legal scenarios in clinical documentation, healthcare professionals should:

A) Assume common sense is enough to determine the right course of action.

B) Rely solely on their personal judgment in all situations.

C) Understand and comply with relevant healthcare regulations.

D) Avoid consulting legal or ethical guidelines to save time.

10. Documenting decisions to breach confidentiality should include:

A) Only the fact that information was disclosed, without reasons.

B) Detailed personal opinions about the patient.

C) The rationale and specific information disclosed.

D) Fabricated justifications to cover legal bases.

Answers:

1. C) Both A and B.

2. B) A patient poses a clear and immediate risk of serious harm to others.

3. A) Ignoring ethical principles to expedite care.

4. B) Communicable diseases with public health risks.

5. C) Various ethical principles, professional standards, and patient interests.

6. B) Explaining how patient information will be used and shared.

7. C) Preventing significant harm to the patient or others.

8. B) Parents or legal guardians.

9. C) Understand and comply with relevant healthcare regulations.

10. C) The rationale and specific information disclosed.

Chapter 13: The Future of Clinical Documentation

13.1 Emerging Trends and Technologies

The landscape of clinical documentation is rapidly evolving, driven by advances in technology and changing healthcare delivery models. These innovations aim to enhance the efficiency, accuracy, and patient-centeredness of documentation, ultimately improving patient care and healthcare outcomes. This section explores key emerging trends and technologies shaping the future of clinical documentation.

Artificial Intelligence (AI) and Natural Language Processing (NLP)

- AI and NLP are transforming clinical documentation by automating the transcription of clinical encounters and extracting meaningful data from unstructured text. This technology can significantly reduce the documentation burden on healthcare providers, allowing more time for patient care.

- AI-powered tools are also being developed to assist with clinical decision-making by providing insights and recommendations based on the analysis of vast amounts of clinical data.

Voice Recognition Software

- Voice recognition technology enables healthcare providers to dictate clinical notes directly into electronic health records (EHRs), improving the speed and convenience of documentation. Ongoing advancements are increasing the accuracy and reliability of voice recognition, making it a valuable tool for clinical documentation.

Interoperable Electronic Health Records (EHRs)

- The push for EHR interoperability aims to enable seamless data exchange between different healthcare systems and providers. This ensures that comprehensive patient information is accessible across the continuum of care, enhancing coordination and the quality of care provided.

- Interoperability standards, such as Fast Healthcare Interoperability Resources (FHIR), are facilitating this integration by providing a framework for the exchange of healthcare information electronically.

Telehealth and Remote Patient Monitoring

- The expansion of telehealth services, accelerated by global health challenges, has necessitated innovations in documentation practices to accommodate virtual patient encounters. Remote patient monitoring technologies also contribute data directly to EHRs, providing real-time insights into patients' health status outside of traditional clinical settings.

- Documentation tools integrated with telehealth platforms are evolving to capture the nuances of virtual care delivery, ensuring that telehealth encounters are documented with the same rigor as in-person visits.

Patient-Generated Health Data (PGHD)

- With the proliferation of wearable devices and health apps, patients are increasingly generating health data outside of clinical settings. Integrating PGHD into clinical documentation provides a more comprehensive view of the patient's health and lifestyle, supporting personalized and preventive care.

- Strategies for securely incorporating PGHD into EHRs are being developed, along with guidelines for interpreting and acting on this data.

Blockchain in Healthcare

- Blockchain technology is being explored for its potential to securely manage health records, ensuring data integrity and patient control over their information. By providing a secure, decentralized platform for health data, blockchain could revolutionize how patient information is stored, shared, and protected.

Conclusion

The future of clinical documentation is characterized by technological innovation and a shift towards more patient-centered, efficient, and data-driven healthcare delivery. As these emerging trends and technologies continue to evolve, they offer the promise of transforming clinical documentation processes, improving healthcare outcomes, and enhancing the patient care experience. Adapting to these changes will require ongoing education, flexibility, and collaboration among healthcare professionals, technology developers, and policymakers.

13.2 The Evolution of Documentation Standards

The standards governing clinical documentation have evolved significantly over the years, reflecting changes in healthcare delivery, regulatory requirements, and technological advancements. This evolution aims to improve the quality, safety, and efficiency of patient care, as well as to enhance communication among healthcare providers and between providers and patients. As we look to the future, it's clear that documentation standards will continue to adapt in response to new challenges and opportunities. Here's an overview of how documentation standards have evolved and where they might be headed.

Historical Perspective

- **Paper-Based Records**: Traditionally, clinical documentation was entirely paper-based, leading to challenges with storage, accessibility, and legibility. Standards were focused on ensuring comprehensive and clear documentation within these physical records.

- **Introduction of Electronic Health Records (EHRs)**: The shift to EHRs marked a significant change in documentation practices, emphasizing the need for standardized data entry fields, templates, and coding systems to ensure consistency and enable data sharing.

Current Trends

- **Interoperability Standards**: With the adoption of EHRs, a major focus has been on developing and implementing interoperability standards (e.g., HL7, FHIR) to facilitate the seamless exchange of healthcare information across different systems and settings.

- **Data Privacy and Security**: The increasing digitization of health records has brought data privacy and security to the forefront, with standards and regulations (e.g., HIPAA, GDPR) being developed to protect patient information.

- **Quality and Outcome-Based Documentation**: Recent standards emphasize not just the quantity of documentation but its quality, with a focus on accurately reflecting patient outcomes, care coordination, and adherence to evidence-based practices.

Future Directions

- **Incorporation of Artificial Intelligence (AI) and Machine Learning (ML)**: As AI and ML technologies become more integrated into healthcare, documentation standards will need to address the use of these tools for generating and reviewing clinical notes, ensuring accuracy, and maintaining transparency in automated processes.

- **Patient-Centered Documentation**: Standards will increasingly emphasize the importance of documenting patient preferences, goals, and shared decision-making processes, reflecting a shift towards more patient-centered care models.

- **Global Harmonization**: As healthcare becomes more globally interconnected, there will be a push towards harmonizing documentation standards across countries to support international research, telehealth, and patient care.

- **Real-Time and Predictive Documentation**: Advancements in technology will enable more real-time documentation of patient encounters and the use of predictive analytics to guide care planning, requiring standards that support these dynamic uses of clinical data.

Challenges and Considerations

- **Balancing Innovation with Usability**: As documentation standards evolve to incorporate new technologies, maintaining usability for healthcare providers to prevent increased administrative burden will be crucial.

- **Ensuring Equity**: Ensuring that documentation standards do not inadvertently create or exacerbate healthcare disparities is important, particularly as technologies like AI are integrated into healthcare practices.

Conclusion

The evolution of documentation standards is an ongoing process that reflects broader trends in healthcare, technology, and society. By staying informed and adaptable, healthcare providers can navigate these changes, contributing to the development of documentation practices that enhance patient care, improve outcomes, and meet the needs of an increasingly complex healthcare environment.

13.3 Preparing for the Future of Healthcare

The future of healthcare is poised to be shaped by rapid advancements in technology, shifts in patient care models, and evolving healthcare needs. As such, preparing for the future is not just about adopting new technologies but also about embracing changes in how healthcare is delivered and how patient care is documented and managed. Here's a comprehensive approach to gearing up for the forthcoming transformations in healthcare.

Embracing Technological Innovations

- **Stay Informed**: Keep abreast of emerging technologies such as artificial intelligence (AI), machine learning (ML), blockchain, and telehealth that are set to transform healthcare delivery and documentation.

- **Invest in Training**: Ensure that healthcare professionals are well-trained in utilizing new technologies and understand their implications for clinical practice and documentation.

- **Evaluate and Adapt**: Regularly assess new technologies for their potential to improve patient care and operational efficiency. Be prepared to adapt workflows and documentation practices to integrate these innovations effectively.

Fostering a Culture of Lifelong Learning

- **Continuous Education**: Encourage a culture of continuous learning within healthcare organizations. Provide opportunities for healthcare professionals to update their knowledge and skills through professional development programs and continuous education.

- **Interdisciplinary Collaboration**: Promote collaboration between different healthcare disciplines to foster a holistic understanding of patient care and documentation requirements. This can lead to more comprehensive care and innovative approaches to healthcare challenges.

Enhancing Patient-Centered Care

- **Patient Engagement**: Engage patients as active participants in their care. Utilize patient portals and digital tools to enhance communication, provide access to health information, and involve patients in decision-making processes.

- **Personalized Care**: Leverage data analytics and precision medicine to tailor treatments to individual patient needs, preferences, and genetic profiles. Documentation practices should reflect this personalized approach to care.

Adapting to Changing Healthcare Landscapes

- **Regulatory Compliance**: Stay updated on changes in healthcare regulations and standards. Ensure that documentation practices comply with current legal and ethical requirements.

- **Global Health Considerations**: Recognize the increasing importance of global health considerations, including the need for preparedness for pandemics and the integration of global health data. Documentation practices may need to adapt to these broader health contexts.

Prioritizing Data Security and Privacy

- **Strengthen Security Measures**: As healthcare increasingly relies on digital platforms, prioritizing the security and privacy of patient data is critical. Implement robust cybersecurity measures and educate staff on data protection practices.

- **Transparency and Trust**: Maintain transparency with patients about how their data is used and protected. Building trust is essential for effective patient engagement and the successful implementation of new technologies.

Conclusion

Preparing for the future of healthcare requires a multifaceted approach that embraces technological innovation, promotes lifelong learning, enhances patient-centered care, and adapts to changing healthcare environments. By anticipating these changes and proactively planning for them, healthcare providers can ensure they are well-positioned to meet the challenges and opportunities of the future, ultimately leading to improved patient care and health outcomes.

13.4 Exercise: 10 MCQs with Answers at the End

Let's create a set of 10 multiple-choice questions (MCQs) based on the content of Chapter 13, focusing on emerging trends and technologies, the evolution of documentation standards, preparing for the future of healthcare, and the overall theme of advancements in clinical documentation. This exercise aims to reinforce key concepts and assess understanding.

1. Which technology is transforming clinical documentation by automating transcription and extracting meaningful data?

  A) Blockchain

  B) Artificial Intelligence (AI) and Natural Language Processing (NLP)

  C) Virtual Reality (VR)

  D) 3D Printing

2. Voice recognition software in clinical documentation improves:

  A) Only the security of patient data

  B) The speed and convenience of documentation

  C) The accuracy of billing processes exclusively

  D) The physical storage needs for records

3. The push for EHR interoperability aims to:

  A) Limit access to patient records

  B) Enable seamless data exchange between different healthcare systems

  C) Reduce the use of digital health records

D) Increase the complexity of healthcare data management

4. Patient portals contribute to patient engagement by providing:

A) Access to the latest medical research only

B) Secure online access to health records and information

C) Entertainment through health-related games

D) A platform for healthcare professionals to share insights

5. Blockchain technology in healthcare is being explored for:

A) Reducing the need for patient consent

B) Managing health records with enhanced security and patient control

C) Decreasing transparency in health data management

D) Eliminating electronic health records (EHRs)

6. An important consideration in the evolution of documentation standards is:

A) The return to paper-based records for their reliability

B) Balancing innovation with usability to prevent increased administrative burden

C) Avoiding the use of standardized terminologies to maintain diversity

D) Phasing out all digital documentation tools to protect patient privacy

7. Preparing for the future of healthcare involves all EXCEPT:

A) Ignoring technological innovations that could disrupt traditional practices

B) Investing in training for healthcare professionals on new technologies

C) Fostering a culture of continuous learning within healthcare organizations

D) Engaging patients as active participants in their care

8. The incorporation of artificial intelligence in healthcare aims to:

A) Replace all human decision-making in patient care

B) Support clinical decision-making by providing insights from large datasets

C) Discourage interdisciplinary collaboration in clinical settings

D) Simplify healthcare to basic algorithms, eliminating the need for specialists

9. Adapting to changing healthcare landscapes requires:

A) Decreased focus on regulatory compliance and global health considerations

B) Enhanced collaboration across different healthcare disciplines

C) A shift away from patient-centered care models to reduce complexity

D) The exclusion of precision medicine and data analytics in care planning

10. A critical aspect of preparing for the future of healthcare is:

A) Prioritizing data security and privacy with robust cybersecurity measures

B) Limiting patient access to digital health tools to maintain traditional roles

C) Focusing solely on in-person care models and avoiding telehealth

D) Reducing investments in continuous education and professional development

Answers:

1. B) Artificial Intelligence (AI) and Natural Language Processing (NLP)

2. B) The speed and convenience of documentation

3. B) Enable seamless data exchange between different healthcare systems

4. B) Secure online access to health records and information

5. B) Managing health records with enhanced security and patient control

6. B) Balancing innovation with usability to prevent increased administrative burden

7. A) Ignoring technological innovations that could disrupt traditional practices

8. B) Support clinical decision-making by providing insights from large datasets

9. B) Enhanced collaboration across different healthcare disciplines

10. A) Prioritizing data security and privacy with robust cybersecurity measures

Chapter 14: Case Studies and Real-World Applications

14.1 Analyzing Successful Documentation Strategies

This section explores real-world examples of successful documentation strategies implemented by healthcare organizations. By examining these case studies, we can identify key factors contributing to their success and learn how to apply these strategies to improve clinical documentation in various healthcare settings.

Case Study 1: Implementing an AI-powered Documentation Assistant

Background: A large hospital system faced challenges with the administrative burden on clinicians, leading to documentation burnout and reduced time for patient care. To address this, the hospital implemented an AI-powered documentation assistant integrated with their EHR system.

Strategy: The AI assistant used natural language processing (NLP) to transcribe clinician-patient conversations during visits and automatically populate the EHR with relevant clinical notes.

Clinicians could review and edit these notes, ensuring accuracy while significantly reducing manual documentation time.

Outcomes:

- Reduced documentation time by 30%, allowing clinicians more time for patient care.

- Improved documentation accuracy and completeness.

- High clinician satisfaction with the new tool, reducing burnout.

Case Study 2: Enhancing Interoperability for Better Care Coordination

Background: A regional healthcare network struggled with care coordination across its various facilities due to disparate EHR systems. Important patient information was often siloed, hindering efficient care delivery.

Strategy: The network invested in enhancing EHR interoperability using standards like Fast Healthcare Interoperability Resources (FHIR). This allowed for seamless data exchange between facilities, enabling a unified view of patient records.

Outcomes:

- Improved care coordination and patient outcomes, with a notable reduction in duplicative testing.

- Enhanced patient satisfaction due to more cohesive care experiences.

- Increased operational efficiency and reduced costs associated with redundant tests and procedures.

Case Study 3: Utilizing EHR Templates for Standardization

Background: A multi-specialty clinic identified inconsistencies in clinical documentation practices among its providers, affecting the quality of care and compliance with coding and billing requirements.

Strategy: The clinic developed and implemented customized EHR templates for common conditions and procedures. These templates guided providers through the documentation process, ensuring that all necessary information was captured consistently.

Outcomes:

- Increased documentation consistency and compliance with best practices.

- Improved coding accuracy and billing efficiency, resulting in higher reimbursement rates.

- Enhanced quality of care through more comprehensive and standardized documentation.

Key Factors for Successful Documentation Strategies

- **User Engagement**: Involving clinicians and other end-users in the development and implementation of documentation tools ensures that these solutions meet their needs and are more likely to be adopted successfully.

- **Training and Support**: Providing comprehensive training and ongoing support for new documentation practices is crucial for ensuring smooth transitions and maximizing the benefits of these strategies.

- **Continuous Evaluation**: Regularly assessing the impact of documentation strategies on clinical workflows, patient care, and administrative efficiency allows for ongoing optimization.

Conclusion

These case studies highlight the potential of innovative documentation strategies to address common challenges in healthcare settings. By leveraging technology, enhancing interoperability, and standardizing documentation practices, healthcare organizations can improve efficiency, quality of care, and clinician satisfaction. The key to success lies in engaging users, providing adequate training and support, and continuously evaluating and refining documentation practices.

14.2 Learning from Documentation Failures

Analyzing documentation failures provides invaluable lessons for healthcare organizations, enabling them to identify vulnerabilities in their processes and implement strategies to prevent future issues. This section explores case studies where documentation failures led to negative outcomes, underscoring the importance of robust documentation practices in ensuring patient safety and legal compliance.

Case Study 1: Incomplete Documentation Leading to Medication Error

Background: A small hospital experienced a serious medication error when a patient was administered a drug they were allergic to. The allergy information was not documented in the patient's electronic health record (EHR) due to incomplete data entry during the admission process.

Analysis:

- The investigation revealed that the omission was due to the clinician's oversight and the lack of prompts in the EHR system for mandatory allergy documentation.

- The error highlighted the need for comprehensive checks and balances in the documentation process to ensure critical patient information is accurately captured.

Lessons Learned:

- Implement mandatory fields in EHRs for critical patient information such as allergies.

- Conduct regular training for staff on the importance of complete and accurate documentation.

- Introduce regular audits of patient records to identify and rectify documentation gaps.

Case Study 2: Poor Documentation Leading to Legal Action

Background: A healthcare provider faced legal action after a patient suffered complications from a procedure. The provider's defense was compromised by inadequate documentation that failed to accurately reflect the care provided and the informed consent process.

Analysis:

- The documentation did not include detailed notes on the patient's condition before the procedure, the rationale for the chosen treatment, or the discussion of risks and alternatives with the patient.

- This lack of detailed documentation made it difficult to demonstrate that the standard of care was met and that the patient had been properly informed.

Lessons Learned:

- Ensure detailed documentation of the care process, including patient condition, treatment rationale, and informed consent discussions.

- Adopt standardized templates for consent and procedure documentation to ensure all necessary information is consistently recorded.

- Provide ongoing education on legal aspects of clinical documentation and the role of documentation in defending against malpractice claims.

Case Study 3: Miscommunication Due to Inconsistent Documentation

Background: A multidisciplinary team experienced a critical miscommunication regarding a patient's treatment plan due to inconsistent documentation across different sections of the patient's EHR.

Analysis:

- The inconsistency arose from the use of different terminology and treatment plan descriptions by various team members, leading to confusion and the implementation of an incorrect treatment protocol.

- This case underscored the importance of standardized documentation practices and clear communication among the care team.

Lessons Learned:

- Implement standardized documentation practices and terminologies across all disciplines within the healthcare organization.

- Encourage regular interdisciplinary team meetings to discuss patient care plans and ensure consistency in documentation.

- Utilize EHR features such as shared notes or interdisciplinary care plans to facilitate clear and consistent communication among care team members.

Conclusion

Documentation failures can have serious implications for patient safety, legal liability, and the overall quality of care. Learning from these failures is essential for healthcare organizations to enhance their documentation practices, improve patient outcomes, and mitigate risks. Implementing standardized processes, conducting regular training, and fostering clear communication are key strategies to prevent documentation failures.

14.3 Innovations in Clinical Documentation

Innovations in clinical documentation are reshaping the landscape of healthcare, aiming to improve the efficiency of healthcare providers, enhance the quality of patient care, and ensure the security and privacy of patient information. These advancements leverage cutting-edge technologies and methodologies to address traditional challenges in documentation practices. This section highlights several innovations that are setting new standards in clinical documentation.

Speech Recognition and Natural Language Processing (NLP)

Innovation: The integration of speech recognition and NLP technologies into clinical documentation processes enables healthcare providers to dictate notes verbally. These technologies transcribe spoken language into text and can interpret and structure unstructured data into EHR-compatible formats.

Impact:

- **Efficiency**: Significantly reduces the time required for documentation, allowing providers to spend more time on patient care.

- **Accuracy**: Advanced NLP algorithms can understand context and nuances in speech, improving the accuracy of transcribed notes.

Blockchain for Secure and Immutable Records

Innovation: Blockchain technology offers a decentralized approach to storing health records, creating an immutable ledger of patient data that can enhance security and patient control over their information.

Impact:

- **Security**: Provides a secure platform for storing patient records, reducing the risk of data breaches.

- **Patient Empowerment**: Allows patients to control who has access to their information, fostering trust and engagement.

Predictive Analytics and AI-driven Insights

Innovation: Utilizing AI and predictive analytics to analyze vast amounts of clinical data, these tools can identify patterns, predict outcomes, and provide decision support to healthcare providers directly within the documentation workflow.

Impact:

- **Proactive Care**: Enables more proactive and preventive care approaches by identifying at-risk patients early.

- **Personalized Treatment**: Supports personalized treatment plans by analyzing patient data and comparing it with similar cases and evidence-based practices.

Interoperable EHR Systems

Innovation: Advances in EHR interoperability facilitate seamless data exchange across different healthcare systems and providers, ensuring that comprehensive patient information is readily available whenever and wherever it is needed.

Impact:

- **Continuity of Care**: Enhances the continuity of care across different care settings and disciplines.

- **Collaborative Care**: Improves collaborative care planning among multidisciplinary teams.

Patient-Generated Health Data (PGHD) Integration

Innovation: Incorporating PGHD from wearable devices, mobile apps, and home monitoring equipment into clinical documentation provides a more holistic view of the patient's health outside the clinical setting.

Impact:

- **Engagement**: Engages patients in their health management, promoting healthier lifestyles and adherence to treatment plans.

- **Comprehensive Care**: Offers providers a more comprehensive understanding of patient health, supporting more informed decision-making.

Telehealth Documentation Platforms

Innovation: Specialized documentation platforms designed for telehealth streamline the capture and integration of virtual visit information into the patient's primary health record.

Impact:

- **Accessibility**: Expands access to care for patients in remote or underserved areas.

- **Efficiency**: Facilitates the efficient documentation of telehealth encounters, ensuring they are recorded with the same level of detail and accuracy as in-person visits.

Conclusion

The innovations in clinical documentation are driven by the need to address the complexities of modern healthcare delivery, improve patient outcomes, and optimize provider workflows. By embracing these technological advancements, healthcare organizations can overcome traditional documentation challenges, setting a new standard for quality, efficiency, and patient-centered care in the digital age.

14.4 Exercise: 10 MCQs with Answers at the End

Let's create a set of 10 multiple-choice questions (MCQs) based on the content of Chapter 14, focusing on analyzing successful documentation strategies, learning from documentation failures, innovations in clinical documentation, and real-world applications. This exercise aims to reinforce key concepts and assess understanding.

1. What technology has significantly reduced the documentation burden on healthcare providers by transcribing clinician-patient conversations?

  A) Blockchain

  B) Virtual Reality (VR)

  C) Artificial Intelligence (AI) and Natural Language Processing (NLP)

  D) 3D Printing

2. Which of the following is NOT a benefit of enhancing EHR interoperability?

  A) Increased duplicative testing

  B) Improved care coordination

  C) Enhanced patient satisfaction

  D) Reduced costs associated with redundant tests

3. In the context of clinical documentation, what does blockchain technology primarily offer?

A) Increased workload for clinicians

B) A decentralized platform for secure storage of health records

C) A reduction in patient engagement

D) Limitations on data sharing between healthcare providers

4. What is a primary outcome of integrating patient-generated health data (PGHD) into clinical documentation?

A) Decreased patient involvement in healthcare

B) Reduced accuracy of health records

C) A more comprehensive view of the patient's health

D) Increased privacy concerns without benefits

5. Which innovation aims to provide real-time decision support by analyzing clinical data?

A) Predictive analytics and AI-driven insights

B) Wearable fitness trackers

C) Manual paper charting

D) Traditional face-to-face consultations

6. A major challenge identified in a case study of documentation failure was:

A) Overdocumentation of patient encounters

B) Incomplete documentation leading to a medication error

C) Excessive reliance on patient narratives

D) Lack of technology in documenting patient information

7. Successful documentation strategies often include:

A) Avoiding the use of electronic health record (EHR) systems

B) Implementing AI-powered documentation assistants

C) Decreasing interoperability between different healthcare systems

D) Reducing patient access to their own health records

8. A key factor for successful implementation of new documentation technologies is:

A) Limiting training and support for healthcare professionals

B) Engaging only senior physicians in the decision-making process

C) Regularly assessing the impact on clinical workflows and patient care

D) Increasing the complexity of documentation processes

9. Speech recognition technology in clinical documentation improves:

  A) Only the physical storage needs for records

  B) The security of patient data exclusively

  C) The speed and convenience of documentation

  D) The accuracy of billing processes only

10. Preparing for the future of healthcare documentation requires all EXCEPT:

  A) Embracing technological innovations

  B) Ignoring global health considerations

  C) Investing in continuous education and training

  D) Prioritizing data security and privacy

Answers:

1. C) Artificial Intelligence (AI) and Natural Language Processing (NLP)

2. A) Increased duplicative testing

3. B) A decentralized platform for secure storage of health records

4. C) A more comprehensive view of the patient's health

5. A) Predictive analytics and AI-driven insights

6. B) Incomplete documentation leading to a medication error

7. B) Implementing AI-powered documentation assistants

8. C) Regularly assessing the impact on clinical workflows and patient care

9. C) The speed and convenience of documentation

10. B) Ignoring global health considerations

Chapter 15: Building a Career as a Clinical Documentation Specialist

15.1 Pathways to Becoming a Documentation Specialist

A career as a clinical documentation specialist (CDS) offers an opportunity to play a crucial role in healthcare delivery by ensuring accurate, timely, and compliant medical documentation. This field requires a unique blend of medical knowledge, understanding of healthcare regulations, and skills in health information technology. Here's how to embark on this rewarding career path.

Educational Foundations

- **Bachelor's Degree**: Although requirements can vary, a bachelor's degree in health information management, nursing, or a related healthcare field is often recommended. These programs provide a solid foundation in medical terminology, anatomy, physiology, and healthcare systems.

- **Certifications and Specializations**: Pursuing certifications such as the Certified Clinical Documentation Specialist (CCDS) or the

Certified Documentation Improvement Practitioner (CDIP) can enhance employability and credibility in the field. Specializations in areas like coding and health informatics can also be beneficial.

Gaining Relevant Experience

- **Healthcare Experience**: Prior experience in nursing, medical coding, or health information management can provide valuable insights into patient care processes and documentation requirements.

- **Internships and Entry-Level Positions**: Internships or entry-level roles in medical records departments or health information management can offer hands-on experience with EHR systems and documentation practices.

Developing Essential Skills

- **Attention to Detail**: Accuracy is paramount in clinical documentation, as it directly impacts patient care and billing processes.

- **Analytical Skills**: The ability to analyze patient records and identify documentation gaps or areas for improvement is critical.

- **Communication Skills**: Effective communication with healthcare providers is necessary to clarify documentation and ensure it accurately reflects patient care.

- **Technical Proficiency**: Familiarity with EHR systems and proficiency in navigating and managing digital health records are essential.

Continuing Education and Networking

- **Ongoing Learning**: Healthcare regulations and technologies are constantly evolving. Engaging in continuous education through workshops, conferences, and online courses can keep a documentation specialist up-to-date.

- **Professional Organizations**: Joining professional organizations such as the Association of Clinical Documentation Improvement Specialists (ACDIS) or the American Health Information Management Association (AHIMA) can provide networking opportunities, resources, and updates on industry standards.

Career Advancement Opportunities

- **Leadership Roles**: Experienced documentation specialists can advance to leadership positions, overseeing documentation improvement programs and teams.

- **Consulting and Education**: Opportunities exist for seasoned specialists to work as consultants, helping healthcare organizations optimize their documentation processes, or as educators, training the next generation of documentation professionals.

The Role of Technology

- As technology continues to influence healthcare documentation, specialists should be prepared to adapt to new tools and systems, such as AI-driven documentation assistants and advanced data analytics platforms.

Conclusion

Building a career as a clinical documentation specialist requires a combination of education, experience, and skills development. By staying informed about advancements in healthcare technology and regulations, and continuously improving their knowledge and skills, individuals can thrive in this dynamic and essential field. The pathway to becoming a documentation specialist is marked by opportunities for growth, specialization, and making a significant impact on healthcare quality and efficiency.

15.2 Key Skills and Attributes for Success

A career as a clinical documentation specialist (CDS) is both challenging and rewarding, requiring a unique set of skills and attributes to ensure success. These professionals play a critical role in the healthcare system, enhancing the quality and accuracy of medical records to support patient care, billing, and regulatory compliance. Here are key skills and attributes that are essential for anyone looking to excel in this field.

Clinical Knowledge

- **Understanding of Medical Terminology and Procedures**: A strong foundation in medical terminology, anatomy, physiology, and pharmacology is essential for interpreting clinical scenarios and accurately documenting patient care.

- **Familiarity with Healthcare Practices**: Knowledge of clinical pathways, standards of care, and treatment protocols enables CDS professionals to identify gaps in documentation and suggest improvements.

Analytical Skills

- **Critical Thinking**: The ability to analyze patient records, identify inconsistencies or missing information, and understand the implications for patient care and billing is crucial.

- **Problem-Solving**: Effective CDS professionals are adept at finding solutions to documentation challenges, ensuring that records fully capture the patient's clinical status and care provided.

Communication Skills

- **Interpersonal Communication**: Strong verbal and written communication skills are necessary for interacting with physicians, nurses, and other healthcare professionals to clarify and improve documentation.

- **Educational Abilities**: The capacity to educate healthcare staff about documentation practices, coding guidelines, and regulatory requirements is important for promoting consistent and compliant documentation across the organization.

Technological Proficiency

- **EHR Systems**: Proficiency with electronic health record (EHR) systems is a must, as these are the primary tools for documenting patient care.

- **Adaptability to New Technologies**: With the rapid advancement of technology in healthcare, being adaptable and open to learning new systems and tools is essential.

Attention to Detail

- Precision is key in clinical documentation. Small details can have significant implications for patient care, billing, and legal matters. CDS professionals must ensure that all aspects of patient encounters are accurately recorded.

Ethical Standards and Integrity

- **Confidentiality**: Maintaining patient privacy and adhering to laws and regulations governing the use and disclosure of health information is paramount.

- **Honesty**: Accuracy in documentation is critical; CDS professionals must uphold high standards of honesty and integrity, ensuring that records reflect the true nature of patient care.

Organizational Skills

- **Time Management**: The ability to manage priorities and work efficiently is important, especially when dealing with multiple cases or tight deadlines.

- **Documentation Management**: Organizing and maintaining records systematically to ensure ease of access and compliance with retention policies.

Professional Development

- **Continuous Learning**: The healthcare field is continuously evolving. Successful CDS professionals commit to lifelong learning to stay updated on the latest in medical science, documentation standards, and regulations.

- **Networking**: Engaging with professional communities and participating in relevant workshops and conferences can provide valuable insights and opportunities for career growth.

Conclusion

The role of a clinical documentation specialist requires a balanced mix of clinical knowledge, analytical and communication skills, technological proficiency, attention to detail, ethical standards, and organizational skills. Cultivating these attributes not only enables success in the field but also significantly contributes to the improvement of healthcare quality and patient outcomes.

15.3 Navigating the Job Market and Career Advancement

Finding success in the job market as a clinical documentation specialist and advancing in this career involves strategic planning, continuous learning, and networking. As healthcare documentation becomes increasingly vital for patient care quality, regulatory compliance, and efficient healthcare delivery, the demand for skilled documentation specialists continues to grow. Here are strategies to navigate the job market and pursue career advancement in this field.

Understanding the Landscape

- **Research the Field**: Begin by understanding the scope of work, key responsibilities, and the impact of documentation specialists in healthcare. This knowledge can guide your career path decisions and help you tailor your skill set to meet industry needs.

- **Stay Informed About Industry Trends**: Keeping abreast of changes in healthcare regulations, documentation technologies, and best practices is crucial. This awareness can make you more competitive in the job market and open up opportunities for advancement.

Building a Strong Foundation

- **Acquire Relevant Education**: Pursuing a degree or certification in health information management, nursing, or a related field can provide a solid foundation. Specialized certifications in documentation improvement can further enhance your qualifications.

- **Gain Practical Experience**: Entry-level positions or internships in medical records departments or health information management can offer hands-on experience. Volunteering in healthcare settings can also provide valuable exposure.

Highlighting Your Skills and Experience

- **Develop a Compelling Resume**: Highlight your clinical knowledge, experience with electronic health record systems, certifications, and any specializations. Emphasize your achievements in improving documentation quality, efficiency, or compliance.

- **Prepare for Interviews**: Be ready to discuss how your skills can address the specific needs of employers, including examples of how you have successfully tackled documentation challenges.

Continuous Learning and Development

- **Pursue Further Education**: Engaging in ongoing education through workshops, seminars, and online courses can keep your skills sharp and relevant. Consider advanced degrees or certifications that can open up higher-level positions.

- **Stay Technologically Savvy**: With the rapid evolution of healthcare technology, proficiency in the latest electronic health record systems and documentation tools is vital. Seek opportunities to learn about new technologies and their application in clinical documentation.

Networking and Professional Involvement

- **Join Professional Organizations**: Membership in professional organizations can provide networking opportunities, access to industry news, and resources for professional development.

Attend conferences and seminars to connect with peers and leaders in the field.

- **Mentorship**: Seek mentorship from experienced professionals in clinical documentation. Mentors can offer guidance, career advice, and introductions to opportunities in the field.

Seeking Advancement Opportunities

- **Demonstrate Leadership**: Take on leadership roles in projects or committees within your organization. Showing initiative and the ability to lead and improve documentation practices can position you for advancement.

- **Consider Specialization or Consulting**: Specializing in areas such as coding, compliance, or health informatics can differentiate you in the job market. Experienced professionals may also find opportunities in consulting, providing expertise to healthcare organizations on documentation improvement initiatives.

Conclusion

Navigating the job market and pursuing career advancement as a clinical documentation specialist requires a combination of education, practical experience, and a proactive approach to professional development. By staying informed about industry trends, continuously enhancing your skills, and actively engaging with the professional community, you can build a rewarding career that contributes significantly to the quality of healthcare delivery.

15.4 Exercise: 10 MCQs with Answers at the End

Let's create a set of 10 multiple-choice questions (MCQs) based on the content of Chapter 15, focusing on pathways to becoming a documentation specialist, key skills and attributes for success, navigating the job market and career advancement, and overarching themes related to building a career in clinical documentation. This exercise aims to reinforce key concepts and assess understanding.

1. A foundational degree for a career as a clinical documentation specialist is often in:

   A) Fine Arts

   B) Health Information Management

   C) Political Science

   D) Literature

2. Which certification is beneficial for a documentation specialist to enhance employability?

   A) Certified Clinical Documentation Specialist (CCDS)

   B) Certified Public Accountant (CPA)

   C) Certified Information Systems Security Professional (CISSP)

   D) Certified Culinary Scientist (CCS)

3. Key skills for a clinical documentation specialist include all EXCEPT:

A) Culinary arts

B) Analytical skills

C) Attention to detail

D) Clinical knowledge

4. Continuous education in clinical documentation is important due to:

A) The static nature of healthcare regulations

B) Decreasing reliance on technology in healthcare

C) Constantly evolving healthcare regulations and technologies

D) The diminishing role of documentation in patient care

5. Effective communication skills in clinical documentation are crucial for:

A) Interacting with celebrities

B) Clarifying and improving documentation with healthcare providers

C) Negotiating contracts in the entertainment industry

D) Teaching yoga classes

6. Networking can be enhanced through involvement in:

   A) Professional cooking forums

   B) Social media challenges unrelated to healthcare

   C) Professional organizations related to clinical documentation

   D) Fantasy sports leagues

7. A strategy for career advancement in clinical documentation is:

   A) Avoiding new technologies

   B) Ignoring feedback on documentation quality

   C) Demonstrating leadership in documentation improvement projects

   D) Limiting professional development to minimize distractions

8. Specializing in areas like health informatics can:

   A) Decrease a specialist's marketability

   B) Differentiate a specialist in the job market

   C) Confine a specialist to entry-level positions

   D) Discourage continuous learning

9. Mentorship in clinical documentation is valuable for:

   A) Learning ancient languages

   B) Obtaining career advice and guidance

C) Improving culinary skills

D) Mastering musical instruments

10. Staying technologically savvy is vital for a clinical documentation specialist because:

A) It helps in personal blogging endeavors

B) Healthcare technology remains unchanged over decades

C) It's a requirement for all hobbies

D) Healthcare documentation technologies are rapidly evolving

Answers:

1. B) Health Information Management

2. A) Certified Clinical Documentation Specialist (CCDS)

3. A) Culinary arts

4. C) Constantly evolving healthcare regulations and technologies

5. B) Clarifying and improving documentation with healthcare providers

6. C) Professional organizations related to clinical documentation

7. C) Demonstrating leadership in documentation improvement projects

8. B) Differentiate a specialist in the job market

9. B) Obtaining career advice and guidance

10. D) Healthcare documentation technologies are rapidly evolving

Conclusion

As we conclude this comprehensive exploration of clinical documentation, it's clear that this field is integral to the healthcare system. From enhancing patient care and ensuring compliance with healthcare regulations to embracing technological advancements and fostering professional development, the role of clinical documentation specialists is multifaceted and evolving.

We've delved into the importance of accurate and timely documentation, the challenges and innovations shaping the field, and the pathways for those interested in building a career as a documentation specialist. Key takeaways include the necessity of continuous learning, the impact of technology on documentation practices, and the critical role of communication and collaboration in delivering high-quality healthcare.

For individuals looking to enter or advance in this field, the journey involves acquiring a solid educational foundation, gaining relevant experience, and continuously updating skills to stay abreast of industry changes. Success as a clinical documentation specialist not only contributes to the individual's professional growth but also significantly impacts patient outcomes and the efficiency of healthcare delivery.

As healthcare continues to evolve, the demand for skilled documentation specialists will remain strong, highlighting the ongoing need for dedicated professionals committed to excellence in clinical documentation. By adhering to best practices, embracing innovation, and prioritizing patient-centered care, documentation specialists can continue to play a crucial role in the future of healthcare.

*The best way to thank an author is
to
write a review.*